CHARGED PARTICLES (e±) EXCITATION OF NOBLE GASES

KESHAV RAM VERMA

Charged Particles Excitation Of noble gases

First Edition September 2024

Copyright © 2024 Keshav Ram Verma

Written by Keshav Ram Verma

CONTENTS

CHAPTER - 1

INTRODUCTION

1.1 SILENT FEATURES OF ATOMIC SCATTERING

In general, term 'scattering' means a random distribution of certain items by a suitable target. Since scattering occurs due to collision of projectile and scatterer, hence scattering theory is also known as collision theory. Scattering theory is a framework for studying and understanding the fundamental to the branches of physics and astrophysics. It is initiated through the interactions between the electrons and atoms, positron and atoms, neutron and atoms or any other projectile over an appropriate target. In it deviation of particle (projectile) from its original direction is caused by the interaction with the target (scatterer). A large number of parameters defined, are determined in scattering giving the knowledge about forces, structure and charge distribution *etc* of the target because usually the nature of the particle used as projectile is known.

Nearly a century has been passed since the first successful investigation in this field by Rutherford's findings that atom have their mass and positive charge concentrated in almost point like nuclei. Recent discoveries of scattering on smaller lengthy scale and computer simulated theories have made possible that protons and neutrons *etc* are themselves made up of apparently point like quarks. In scattering, one customarily studies collisions among nuclear, sub-nuclear, atomic or molecular particles, and as these are intrinsically quantum systems. It is logical that quantum mechanics is used as the basis for modern scattering theory. Experimental results are used to validate physical and mathematical modeling by a number of exemplary illustrations and comparing theoretical and experimental results. The scattering experiments were rare in physics before quantum mechanics. After quantum mechanics, scattering experiments became the principal method for the study of atoms, molecules and nuclei, since the properties of the scattering system are reflected in the scattering process. The earliest were the alpha-particle scattering experiments that revealed the atomic nucleus. The study of electrical discharges and thermionic vacuum tubes had made available methods of creating high vacuum that are necessary for scattering experiments. The collisions of electrons with atoms are studied extensively, and then the collisions of artificially accelerated nuclear particles-protons, deuterons, neutrons and so on with each other and with nuclei. Therefore scattering is still the primary experimental resource for studying fundamental particles.

The basic scenario is to shoot in a stream of particles, all at the same energy, and detect how many are deflected into detector which measure angles of deflection. We assume all the ingoing particles are represented by wave packets of the same shape and size, so we solve Schrödinger's equation for such a wave packet and find the probability amplitudes for outgoing waves in different directions. We use the term 'particle' only to differentiate from the scattering theory of electromagnetic and mechanical waves, which requires a very different treatment. 'Particle' refers to electrons, positrons, atoms, nuclei and so on. The wave scattering can have particle aspects at high energies (photons), as in Compton scattering, but for this relativity is essential. In collision experiment a number of effects may appear like the elastic, inelastic and super elastic scattering. In elastic scattering the projectile beam of charged particles is scattered in such a way that there is no energy transfer from projectile to internal energy of target. In an inelastic scattering, a part of projectile energy is transferred to internal energy of the target. Further, on the basis of internal motion, inelastic scattering may be classified into two categories. Firstly, the inelastic scattering involves excitation of distinct atomic states. Secondly, the ionizing inelastic collisions involve energy of the electron ejected from target atom. In super elastic scattering the electron gains the energy from internal motion of the atom. It occurs only between an electron and an excited atom.

1.1.1 IDEA OF SCATTERING

In the development of physics, scattering experiments have provided much of our knowledge regarding the forces and interactions in atom and nuclei and hence about the material under certain circumstances. The scattering processes have established most of what we know about the microworld. The study of way of scattering is broadly categorized into two; the classical theory and relativistic quantum theory. In the era of microscopic study, the classical approach is outdated but quantum theory provides basic for relativistic quantum theory, this is why we are presenting little about both approaches.

CLASSICAL THEORY OF SCATTERING

In scattering experiment, a collimated, homogeneous, monoenergetic beam of particles strike the target (scatterer). The intensity of beam is assumed low enough to ignore the mutual interactions of the incident particles and large enough to have good statistics. The target consisting of macroscopic, individual centers is assumed so far as to ignore the coherence effects. After the scattering, particles are detected at a large distance from the target. Assuming the direction of incidence of the beam as Z axis, consider a cone (of solid angle $d\Omega$) oriented at polar and azimuthal angle θ & ϕ respectively, centered at the target.

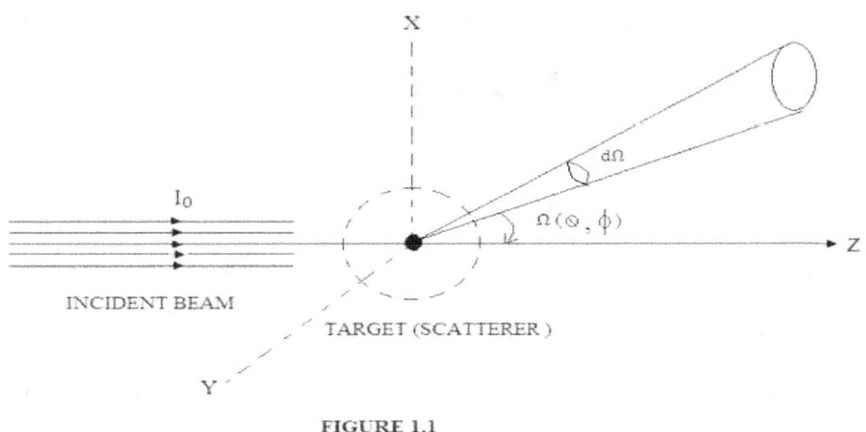

FIGURE 1.1

The number of scattered particles into solid angle $d\Omega$ about set of angle θ & ϕ in unit time is

$$dN \;\propto\; I_0 \, d\Omega$$

or $\qquad dN = \sigma(\theta,\phi) \, I_0 \, d\Omega$ $\qquad\qquad\qquad\qquad\qquad$ .... (1.1)

where $\sigma(\theta,\phi)$ is defined as differential cross section and I_0 is the incident flux density. This differential cross section is simply equal to size of area which, when placed at right angle to the incident beam, would be transversed by many particles as are scattered into unit solid angle around θ and ϕ .

Total scattering cross section is given by

$$\sigma_T = \int \sigma(\theta,\phi) \, d\Omega = \int_{\phi=0}^{2\pi} \int_{\theta=0}^{\pi} \sigma(\theta,\phi) \sin\theta \; d\theta \; d\phi \qquad\qquad .... (1.2)$$

The differential and total cross sections could be regarded as main experimental quantities of the scattering problem. The aim of scattering theory is to make use of these to deduce information or interaction responsible for scattering. Above formulae given by equations (1.1) and (1.2) cease to have meaning when de-Broglie wavelength of the incident particle is appreciable in comparison of dimension of scatterer. In such situation quantum theory of scattering is applicable.

QUANTUM THEORY OF SCATTERING

The simplest model of quantum scattering theory is given by solving the Schrodinger's equation for plane wave impinging on a localized potential. Let $V(r)$ is the potential that a projectile particle encounters due to the target. All the outgoing particles may be represented by a wave packet using the de Broglie's concept. So, we should solve the Schrodinger time dependent equation for such a wave packet. But we adopt a simpler approach of scattering theory in which whole of the system is stationary *i.e.* time independent for a period of time. Thus scattering problem is well approximated by solving Schrodinger's time independent wave equation with an outgoing plane wave.

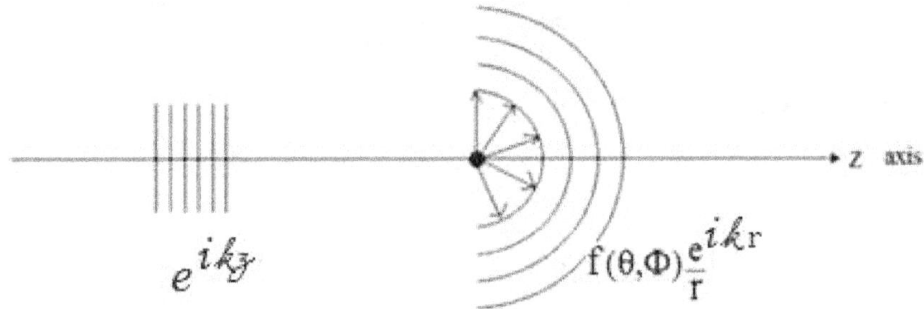

FIGURE 1.2

The Schrodinger time independent wave equation is

$$\nabla^2\Psi + \frac{2m}{\hbar^2}[E - V(r)]\Psi = 0 \qquad\qquad \text{.... (1.3)}$$

Here we shall limit our self to potential $V(r)$ which tends to zero more rapidly than $\frac{1}{r}$ as $r \to \infty$ i.e.

$$\lim_{r\to\infty} r\, V(r) = 0 \qquad\qquad \text{.... (1.4)}$$

Under above circumstance of incoming wave e^{ikz} along Z-direction, in the asymptotic region, the scattered wave function must have the form

$$\Psi = e^{ikz} + f(\theta,\phi)\frac{1}{r}\, e^{ikr} \qquad\qquad \text{.... (1.5)}$$

Here θ & ϕ are measured with respect to incoming wave and $f(\theta,\phi)$ have the dimension of length. The fraction of the beam scattered in a small solid angle $d\Omega$ in a direction (θ,ϕ) through unit area perpendicular to ingoing beam is $\frac{\hbar k}{m}|f(\theta,\phi)|^2 d\Omega$. This in terms gives

Scattering cross section $\quad \sigma(\theta, \phi) = |f(\theta, \phi)|^2$ $\qquad$ .... (1.6)

Total scattering cross section $\quad \sigma_T = \int_\Omega |f(\theta, \phi)|^2 \, d\Omega$ $\qquad$ .... (1.7)

1.1.2 NEED OF ATOMIC SCATTERING IN SCIENCE AND TECHNOLOGY

The atomic collision process involving the charged particles with target atoms is of great interest because there is an increasing demand of the collision cross sections in related field of physics such as astrophysics, laser physics, controlled fusion research, surface science and space science *etc.* Optical emission diagnostics of rare gas plasma are widely used in laboratory and industrial applications [1]. The basic parameters of plasma such as electron temperature and electron density, as well as information about plasma constituents, can be obtained by collisional radiative models [2]. These models require accurate electron excitation cross section data from both the ground and excited states of rare gas atoms, and thus there is need for such cross sectional data over a wide range of projectile energies and for transition between different fine structure levels. The plasma processing of microelectronic structure promises to be a cost effective way of increasing component density and hence the speed and capability of a wide range of devices, *e.g.* in the continued development of plasma deposition, important to economic solar cells and high temperature superconductor development. In magnetically confined fusion machines low temperature plasma occur near the walls of the device. It is essential to understand how wall materials erode and how the resulting impurities are transported to the central plasma region. It is known that line radiation from incompletely stripped atoms can lead to radiation losses and possible prevention of energy break even condition in plasma. Also, the development of new techniques and electronics enables a new generation of experiments to be carried out. The studies on collision processes provide an important landmark for observing the interaction of colliding particles with another. The analysis of such observations leads to an understanding of the various processes resulting from collisions. The electron atom interaction plays an important role in the atmosphere due to impact of charged particles of solar and cosmic origin with the atmospheric constituents. The atomic collision processes control the composition of upper and lower atmosphere and also provide good understanding about the ozone layer depletion. Positron atom scattering involves matter-antimatter interaction. Thus it plays a key role in understanding of many different areas of science and technology. Further the electron atom scattering is one of the fundamental reactions in the atomic physics. The modeling of a non equilibrium plasma requires detailed knowledge of cross section for collision of its components–electrons and atoms, depending on the temperature. To understand the observed characteristic of spectral plasmas and composition of upper and lower atmosphere, the ground state of even nuclei is much useful. It also provides useful information about the ozone layer. It is important in the determination of charge balance and transport properties of electron in low temperature gases and plasma. The range of collision data required is quite wide since almost any charge state of atom is of vital interest. The study of atomic physics provides the most powerful means available for solving the number of unsolved mysteries in the area of astronomy and astrophysics. It is the main objective of astronomical spectroscopy to determine characteristics and physical condition of emitting plasma. Various parameters can be estimated from line intensities, profiles and wavelength of the observed spectral lines. These include the chemical abundance of the elements, the density, temperature and size of emitted region. The interpretation of the observed spectra however is very complicated because of non equilibrium conditions, *e.g.* density may have gradient and excitation of atoms are not in thermodynamically equilibrium at local temperature. Such condition requires a thorough study of atomic data for several physical processes to be available to properly interpret the observed spectra from heavy targets. Therefore, the interpretation of observation data depends on availability and quantity of atomic data in the form of energy levels, transition probabilities, excitation cross sections *etc*. With the advance computer codes, it now becomes possible to obtain accurate atomic data and unravel the mysteries of astronomy.

In condensed matter physics, it provides useful information about the surface and near surface characterization and material modifications. Further one can study the effect of orbital collision by application of external pressure on solids. It is well observed that elastic properties of the materials, *e.g.* elastic constants are varying with temperature and pressure. The scattering process at low temperature plays an important role in many critical applications.

In past few years interaction of intense laser field with atoms is an attractive area of research because it covers a wide range of problems from very basic to applied. Very recently there has been much interest in observation of interference effect, photoemission *etc.* in the interaction of intense laser field with atomic systems. An attractive feature of these studies is that the atomic interference can be controlled by the parameter of the driving field and high harmonic generation. This aspect of controlling atomic response is interesting from both basic and applied point of view. A worldwide resurgence in atomic physics research began in the late 1950 due to its compelling importance to the modeling and diagnostics of plasma germans to other fields of science and to the national programs such as defense or controlled fusion. Very significant process has been made in developing the requisite understanding during the past four decades both experimentally and theoretically but much remain to be done.

The study of positron collision processes provide a sensitive test of the approximate methods developed for electron scattering. A comparative study of electron and positron scattering yields useful information about the role of different interaction potential used in collision dynamics. In recent years considerable attention is paid to the development of theory of positron atom collision and it has also taken speed due to experiments performed with positron beams of controllable energy, which have now become available. The additional importance of positron scattering is that it involves interactions of matter with antimatter, which have possible applications in the astrophysical area. Some investigations are the part motivated by the possible analytical applications of positrons which include surface analysis and medical tomography. The fundamental motivation for studying positron scattering from targets is to compare the scattering cross sections to those of the corresponding electron scattering process. The reason is that positrons can annihilate with an electron of the target during the process. The positron interactions with atoms can cause a variety of intriguing phenomena different from those of the electron case. The reason is that positrons can annihilate with an electron of the target during the process. The Coulomb attraction between positrons and electrons makes an enormous difference from the always repulsive interaction between electrons. The polarization potentials are always attractive, drawing positrons and electrons together. A description of the polarization interaction is very sensible because the static potential has the opposite sign to that of the polarization potential. Therefore the positron-atom problem is indeed more difficult to solve than the electron case, making the theoretical task of describing the phenomena more challenging. Technological applications of positrons are numerous and increasing. These include PET (positron emission tomography) [3] to study metabolic processes, and the characterization of materials [4,5], such as low-dielectric constant insulators for chip manufacture. Positrons offer new ways to study a wide range of other phenomena including plasmas [6], atomic clusters and nanoparticles [7], and a new method to ionize molecules, such as those of biological interest, for mass spectrometry [8].

At low energies, electron interactions are characterized by, amongst other things, strong scattering resonances involving the temporary trapping of the projectile in the field of the atom or molecule. These resonances often lead to profound effects on the scattering cross sections and, in some cases; they can enhance scattering rates by orders of magnitude. Measurements of positron interactions, on the other hand, are not so extensive, or advanced, as those for their matter counterpart. Positron scattering experiments have, generally lacked the specificity and accuracy of electron scattering measurements, mainly as a consequence of low beam intensities and/or relatively poor energy resolution. A significant advance in recent years has been the advent of trap-based positron beams which, when combined with new techniques developed for charged particle scattering in large magnetic fields, have enabled many new measurements. For example, the improved energy resolution and sensitivity offered by these techniques have enabled the first absolute scattering measurements for excitation processes in atoms and molecules, including measurements of positronium formation. These techniques promise much new fundamental information on positron interactions with atoms and molecules, including measurements on biologically important molecules, which may have relevance for a deeper understanding of the interactions that underpin diagnostic techniques such as Positron Emission Tomography.

1.1.3 FUNDAMENTAL OF SCATTERING PROCESS

It is convenient to divide the whole energy range of the incident particle into low, intermediate and high energy regions. In the low energy region, the energy of incident particle remains below the ionization threshold. In this energy region, only few channels are open. Hence eigen function expansion methods are used in low energy region. The close coupling approximation (CCA), R-Matrix theory, partial wave analysis, pseudo-state approximation, optical potential method *etc* are the low energy methods. The intermediate energy region is defined as energy region from two to twenty times of the threshold energy. The high energy region extends upward from the intermediate energy region. There is no single method which can be used reasonably and accurately over the entire energy range. From theoretical point of view, the intermediate energy range is most difficult region in the study of electron/ positron-atom scattering. This is because the interaction of a projectile with atom in this intermediate energy range can involve all the three processes *viz*, elastic scattering, excitation and ionization in a matter. Moreover in intermediate energy range perturbation theory is slightly convergent. In high energy range there may be three processes independently. The perturbation theory is rapidly convergent so that if the energy is high enough the First Born approximation is usually, though not always, applicable. Low energy methods in their original form are not suitable for the intermediate and high energy region, because in this energy region a large number of channels are open for scattering and difficulty arises in computing large number of partial wave. So it is better to work with the integral equations rather than differential equations. At high energies the exchange effects can be neglected due to small interaction time.

The various processes in electron-molecule collisions are:

$e^- + M \rightarrow e^- + M$ Elastic scattering

$e^- + M \rightarrow e^- + M^*$ Electronic excitation

$e^- + M(v) \rightarrow e^- + M(v')$ Vibrational excitation

$e^- + M(j) \rightarrow e^- + M(j')$ Rotational excitation

$e^- + M \rightarrow e^- + A + B$ Electron impact dissociation

$e^- + M \rightarrow A^- + B$ Dissociative attachment

$A^- + B \rightarrow e^- + AB$ Associative detachment

$e^- + M \rightarrow M^+ + 2e^-$ Electron impact ionization

When we consider positron scattering by ground state of atomic hydrogen, the following processes occur which tell that what is the difference between positron-atom scattering and electron-atom scattering.

$e^+ + H(1s) \rightarrow e^+ + H(1s)$ Elastic scattering

$e^+ + H(1s) \rightarrow e^+ + H(nlm)$ Inelastic scattering

$e^+ + H(1s) \rightarrow p + \gamma \text{ ray}$ Annihilation

$e^+ + H(1s) \rightarrow P_S(nlm) + p$ Positronium formation

$e^+ + H(1s) \rightarrow e^+ + e^- + p$ Ionization

Due to the unique properties of positrons, the study of their collisions with atoms, molecules and solids is of great interest not only due to the fundamental understanding of interactions between matter and antimatter, but also to the comparisons with the phenomenon observed with other projectiles, such as electrons, protons and anti-protons. This can provide information about the effects on the scattering process of different masses and charges and hence offer a test of different theoretical approximations. For example, the opposite sign of the charge on the positron and electron has significant effects on the collision process. The important electron-electron exchange effect between the incident electron with the target electrons in electron-atom scattering does not exist in positron-atom scattering. The repulsive static interaction between the positron and atom has the same magnitude but opposite sign to the attractive force between the electron and the atom. However, the polarization potential is attractive and of the same magnitude for both positrons and electrons, due to the dependence of the polarization potential on the quadratic form of the charge of the projectile. The repulsive static and attractive polarization interactions between the positron and atom tend to cancel each other and make the overall interaction generally less attractive than that between an electron and the atom. Consequently, at low energies, when polarization effects are most important, total scattering cross sections are usually much smaller for positrons than for electrons, except for alkali atoms for which significant contribution from positronium formation can occur, while this process is absent for electrons. Another consequence of the partial cancellation of the static and polarization potentials is that a positron is much less likely to be bound to an atom than an electron. The opposite sign of the static and polarization potentials also causes the s-wave elastic scattering phase shift to change sign with incident positron energy between 1 eV and 3 eV, where the contribution from S-wave to the total elastic scattering cross section is zero. At sufficiently high projectile energies the polarization and exchange interactions eventually become negligible compared with the static interaction. The same magnitude of the static interaction for positrons and electrons will result in a merging of the corresponding positron and electron atom scattering cross sections at sufficiently high projectile energy.

The absence of exchange in positron-atom scattering is also an important incentive for the study of the low energy positron scattering. It might have been expected that the absence of exchange effects between the incoming projectile and the target electrons would lead to a simpler formulation of the scattering process than the case with electrons. Unfortunately the strong correlation between positrons and electrons due to the attractive electrostatic interaction between them, introduces even bigger challenges to the description of the collision processes. One of the consequences from this correlation is the positronium formation in which the incident positron forms a stable state by capture of one target electron. Then the collision becomes a two-centre problem in which the centers of the atom and the positronium have to be considered simultaneously. Further the targets with two or more electrons give rise to a further complication, namely the exchange effect with the electron in the positronium and the other electron in the ion, as well as within the target.

1.2 COLLISION PARAMETERS IN SCATTERING PROCESS

The calculation of differential cross section and angular correlation parameters in electron and positron impact excitation of atom are subject of much current theoretical as well as experimental interest. These correlation parameters are much useful in probing the details of atomic structure. By comparison with total and differential cross sections, the study of angular correlation parameters provide a much deeper and more detailed insight into the dynamics of collision process. The measurements of these correlation parameters constitute a strong test of the existing theoretical models of collision process. These angular correlation parameters can be divided into scattering and target parameters. The scattering parameters consist of scattering amplitudes and their phase differences. The target parameters relate to the orientation and alignment of collisionally excited atoms.

In the past few years there has been considerable advance in the techniques used for the development of polarized electron sources and polarized atomic targets.

This development has initiated experiments on the study of scattering of polarized electrons, with polarized target. Such a study is very useful as experimental data can lead to a determination of the spin dependent features of the scattering. The dynamics of the collision process is studied by the investigation of the state to state transition amplitudes. The parameterization of their amplitudes facilitates the physical interpretation of the collision process at most fundamental level, such as the shape and orientations charge cloud and role of exchange during various collision processes. Thus deep insight into the collision processes involving charged particles with target atom requires various collision parameters *e.g.* differential and total scattering cross section, angular correlation parameters, spin resolved parameters, spin asymmetry parameters *etc*. In the past, theories of charged particle impact excitation were mainly applied in calculating the integrated cross sections. However it is quite misleading to judge the success of theoretical approach purely on agreement of integrated cross sections with experimental measurements. A better test of theory could be obtained by comparison of the differential cross sections. The dynamics of the collisional excitation of energy transfer is obtained by studying the polarization of correlation studies. The alignment and orientation parameters offer the most sensitive test to the approximation involved in the theory of charged particles scattering from atoms. The alignment is referred to the shape of excited state charge cloud and its direction in space. The orientation gives the angular momentum transferred to the atom during the course of collision which is not possible from measurement of cross section alone. The study of spin dependent features, such as spin resolved orientation and spin asymmetry parameters makes the use of spin state selectivity. In this section, we shall report the various collision parameters and shall discuss the use of these parameters in science and technology.

1.2.1 CONCEPT OF CROSS SECTION

The cross section is used to express the likelihood of interaction between the target and projectile. When particles in the form of a beam are thrown towards a target, the cross section is a hypothetical area measure around the target that represents a surface. When a beam of particles of type **B** strikes a target consisting of particles of type **T**, some of the **B** particles pass directly through the target while others are deflected. Those are deflected, said to interact or collide with the **T** particles. The cross section σ_{BT} is a measure of the effectiveness of the **B-T** interaction. The larger the cross section, the more likely it is that the **B** particles are deflected.

In general, the cross section is the effective area of the collision region. Here is another classical example that illustrates the concept. Suppose that the target **T** is a solid ball of radius **R** and suppose that the beam particles **B** are point-like. A particle **B** will strike the ball if it passes within a distance of R of the center of the ball. The cross section σ_{BT} for this case is the area of a circle of radius R or R^2 .

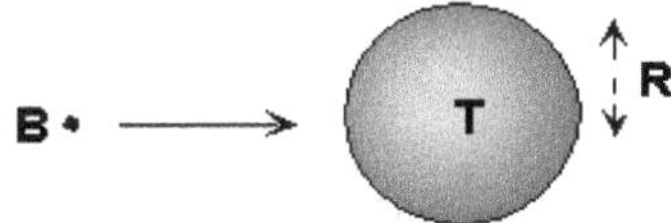

Thus cross section for point-like particles colliding with a sphere is just the area of the sphere projected onto the transverse plane, *i.e.* a circular disk of radius R.

If the beam particles **B** are also balls of radius r, then B is deflected if it comes within a distance of $(R + r)$ from the center of the ball **T**. The cross section σ_{BT} for this case is $\pi(R + r)^2$.

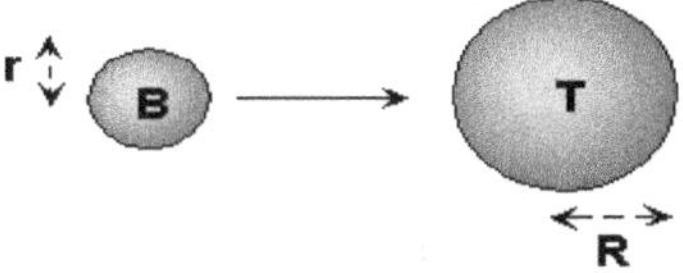

In the microscopic world, elementary particles cannot be considered as ball and they do not interact so mechanically. They can interact at a distance similar to the way two magnets affect each other without touching one another.

To see how this works, return to the macroscopic, mechanical example of a beam of point like **B** particles impinging on target balls **T** of radii R. Suppose that the number of **B** particles per unit volume *i.e.* density of beam particles is n_{beam} and consider that the beam particles are travelling with a speed v. After collision the ball **T** leaves a cylindrical shadow of volume $V = \pi R^2\, v\, t$ in time t.

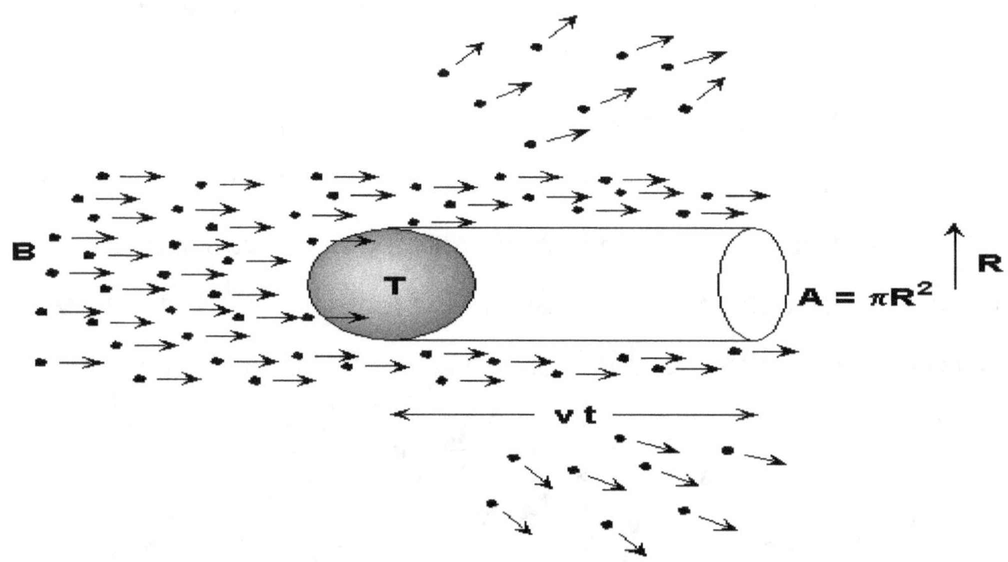

The particles that have been scattered would have been located in the cylinder. The number $N_{interaction}$ of particles that have collided is the number of **B**'s that would be in the 'shadow' region. This number is the volume of the shadow region V times the beam density n_{beam} :

$$N_{interaction} = n_{beam}\, V$$

The number $N_{interactions\ per\ unit\ time}$ of reactions per unit time is

$$\frac{1}{t} N_{interact\ ions\ per\ unit\ time}$$ or

$$N_{interactions\ per\ unit\ time} = n_{beam}\, \pi R^2 V$$

Solving for πR^2, which is the cross section for this particular case, one finds

$$\sigma_{BT} = \frac{N_{interactions\ per\ unit\ time}}{J_{beam}}$$

where J_{beam} is known as the beam flux and is equal to $n_{beam}\, V$. Generally this equation defines the cross section.

Usually the target is consisting of a large number of scattering centre. If N_{target} is the number of particles present in the target then the number of collisions per unit time is N_{target} times greater than the case of a single particle, and one must divide by this factor if the cross section is to represent the effective area of interaction between a single beam particle and a single target particle:

$$\sigma_{BT} = \frac{N_{interactions\ per\ unit\ time}}{J_{beam} \times N_{target}}$$

This is the very basic cross section formula.

1.2.2 DIFFERENTIAL SCATTERING CROSS SECTION AND TOTAL SCATTERING CROSS SECTION

When a beam of energetic electrons passes through a gas, a number of different kinetic processes may result from the encounters of electrons with gas atoms or molecules. These processes can be divided into two categories, inelastic collisions and elastic collisions. The processes involving the loss of kinetic energy by electrons are called inelastic collisions while those involving no loss of kinetic energy by electrons are called elastic collisions. In an inelastic collision, electrons lose kinetic energy owing to the ionization of the target atom, excitation of the target atom, and other internal processes that occur in the atom. In principle, during elastic collisions the electrons lose part of their energy due to momentum transfer, but this energy loss is significantly smaller because it is proportional to the ratio of electron mass to atomic mass.

As a result of the elastic and inelastic collisions, electrons scatter in all directions. The probability of scattering due to either of these two processes can be specified by their respective cross sections. Consider a beam of electrons impinging on target atoms as shown in Figure 1.3. Assume the target particles are at the origin of the coordinate system and the intensity of the incident beam is I. The cross section $d\sigma$ for electrons scattering into a solid angle $d\Omega$ is defined as

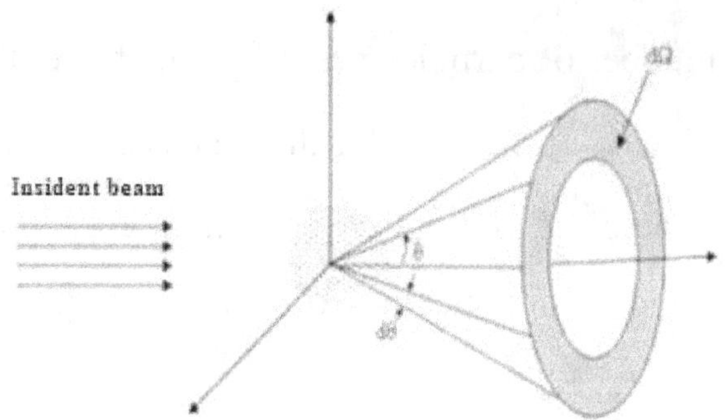

Schematic Diagram of scattering
Figure 1.3

Here the term $d\sigma/d\Omega$ is the differential scattering cross section. It is related to $dN(\theta)$, the number of particles per second scattered into a conical wedge define by θ and $\theta + d\theta$ as follows;

$$\frac{d\sigma}{d\Omega} = \frac{dN(\theta)}{I\,d\Omega}$$ …. (1.8)

The element of solid angle can be written as

$$d\Omega = 2\pi \sin\theta\, d\theta$$ …… (1.9)

where θ is the angle between the scattered and incident directions, known as the scattering angle. For a given process, the total scattering cross section can be defined as

$$\sigma_t = 2\pi \int_0^\pi \frac{d\sigma}{d\Omega} \sin\theta\, d\theta$$ …. (1.10)

1.2.3 ANGULAR CORRELATION PARAMETERS

Fano and Macek [9] have reported the orientation and alignment of the excited atom. According to them, a second rank tensor A and an orientation vector $\vec{O}$ provide significant information about the alignment and the orientation of the excited state for any atom. For an s-p transition Morgan and McDowell [10] have obtained the expression for the orientation and alignment parameters. In terms of the scattering amplitude these are given by

$$
\left.
\begin{aligned}
A_0^c &= \frac{(1-3\lambda)}{2} \\[4pt]
A_{1+}^c &= \frac{\sqrt{2}\,R_e\,\langle a_0 a_1 \rangle}{\sigma} \\[4pt]
A_{2+}^c &= \frac{(\lambda-1)}{2} \\[4pt]
O_{1-}^c &= -\frac{\sqrt{2}\,I_m\,\langle a_0 a_1 \rangle}{\sigma} \\[4pt]
\lambda &= \frac{|a_0|^2}{(|a_0|^2 + 2|a_1|^2)} = \frac{\sigma_0}{\sigma_0 + 2\,\sigma_1} \\[4pt]
\chi &= arg\left(\frac{a_1}{a_0}\right)
\end{aligned}
\right\} \qquad \dots (1.11)
$$

Where a_0 and a_1 are the excitation amplitudes from $m_f = 0$ and $m_f = \pm 1$ magnetic substances, σ_0 and σ_1 are the corresponding differential cross sections. $\sigma = \sigma_0 + 2\sigma_1$ is the total differential cross section summed over all magnetic substances. $<\ >$ denotes the spin averaged value. The parameter χ is the relative phase between the scattering amplitudes a_0 and a_1. It is defined by Eminyan *et al* [11] only when the projections of the system are uniquely fixed or in an approximation where the exchange contribution is neglected.

The orientation parameter is proportional to the expectation value of the angular momentum $< L >$ transferred and the alignment parameter to the mean value of the quadratic expression in L_x, L_y and L_z. Hence the alignment and orientation parameters are also given as

$$
\left.
\begin{aligned}
A_0^c &= \tfrac{1}{2} < 3L_z^2 - L^2 > \\[4pt]
A_{1+}^c &= \tfrac{1}{2} < L_x L_z + L_z L_x > \\[4pt]
A_{2+}^c &= \tfrac{1}{2} < L_x^2 - L_y^2 > \\[4pt]
O_{1-}^c &= \tfrac{1}{2} < L_y >
\end{aligned}
\right\} \qquad \dots (1.12)
$$

Experimentally, the alignment and orientation parameters are measured by using angular correlation experiments in which the angular distribution of the emitted photons is measured in coincidence with the scattered electrons. The measurement of photon angular distribution can provide all information about the alignment of the charge cloud. However, for the determination of the sign of the angular momentum transferred the coherence analysis (*i.e.* the measurement of the circular polarization components) is necessary.

1.2.4 SPIN POLARIZATION PARAMETERS

To understand, the spin polarization parameter, an elementary theory is required.

The Dirac equation for a projectile of rest mass m_0 travelling in central field $V(r)$ at a velocity v is given by

$$[c\boldsymbol{\alpha}.p + \beta m_0 c^2 + V(r)]\psi = E\psi \qquad \text{..... (1.13)}$$

where $E = m_0 \gamma c^2 = E_i + m_0 c^2$ is the total energy, $\gamma = (1 - v^2/c^2)^{-1/2}$, and E_i is the impact kinetic energy of the projectile. The operators $\boldsymbol{\alpha}$ & β in equation (1.13) are usual 4×4 Dirac matrices. The spinor ψ has four components, $\psi = \psi(\psi_1, \psi_2, \psi_3, \psi_4)$, where (ψ_1, ψ_2) are the large components and (ψ_3, ψ_4) are the small components of ψ. For a central potential, the above equation can be reduced to a set of two equations similar to the form of Schrodinger equation as

$$g_l^{\pm''} + \left[K^2 - \frac{l(l+1)}{r^2} - U_l^\pm(r)\right]g_l^\pm(r) = 0 \qquad \text{.... (1.14)}$$

Where $g_l^\pm$ is related to the radial part $G_l^\pm$ of the large component of ψ as

$$G_l = \sqrt{\eta}\,\frac{g_l}{r}, \eta = \frac{[E - V(r) + m_0 c^2]}{c\,\hbar} \quad \& \quad K^2 = \frac{[E^2 - m_0^2 c^4]}{\hbar^2 c^2}$$

The $U_l^\pm$ are the effective Dirac potentials and are given in atomic units ($m_0 = e = \hbar = 1, 1/c = \alpha, where\ \alpha\ is\ the\ fine\ structure\ constant$) as

$$-U_l^+(r) = -2\gamma V + \alpha^2 V^2 - \frac{3}{4}\frac{(\eta')^2}{\eta^2} + \frac{1}{2}\frac{\eta''}{\eta} + \frac{(l+1)}{r}\frac{\eta'}{\eta} \qquad \text{.... (1.15)}$$

and

$$-U_l^-(r) = -2\gamma V + \alpha^2 V^2 - \frac{3}{4}\frac{(\eta')^2}{\eta^2} + \frac{1}{2}\frac{\eta''}{\eta} + \frac{l}{r}\frac{\eta'}{\eta} \qquad \text{.... (1.16)}$$

Till now single and double primes are used corresponding to first and second order derivatives with respect to r, respectively. $\pm$ corresponds to the two eigenvalues of well known spin-orbit interaction, one due to spin up and other due to spin down.

The proper solution of equation (1.14) behaves asymptotically as

$$g_l^\pm(K,r) \simeq Kr\left[j_l(Kr) - \tan\delta_l^\pm n_l(Kr)\right] \qquad \text{.... (1.17)}$$

where j_l and n_l are spherical Bessel functions of the first and second kind, respectively, and $\delta_l^\pm$ are the phase shifts due to collision interactions. The values of $\delta_l^\pm$ may be obtained from equation (1.17). The wave functions $g_l^\pm$ are obtained by numerical integration of equation (1.14) using the Numerov method and the spherical Bessel functions are evaluated as described by N. Sultana et al [12]. C. J. Joachain [13] has given generalized scattering amplitude for the collision process as

$$A = f(K,\theta) + g(K,\theta)\boldsymbol{\sigma}.\hat{\boldsymbol{n}} \qquad \text{..... (1.18)}$$

Here σ is related to spin S as $\sigma = 2S$ and the value of $\langle\boldsymbol{\sigma}.\boldsymbol{L}\rangle$ equals l for $j = l + \frac{1}{2}$ and $-l(l+1)$ for $j = l - \frac{1}{2}$. $f(K,\theta)$ & $g(K,\theta)$ are given

$$f(K,\theta) = \frac{1}{2iK} \sum_{l=0}^{\infty}\left[(l+1)\left(e^{2i\delta_l^+} - 1\right) + l\left(e^{2i\delta_l^-} - 1\right)P_l \cos\theta\right] \qquad \text{.... (1.19a)}$$

$$g(K,\theta) = \frac{1}{2iK} \sum_{l=0}^{\infty}\left[e^{2i\delta_l^+} - e^{2i\delta_l^-}\right]P_l^1 \cos\theta \qquad \text{.... (1.19b)}$$

and $\hat{n}$ is the unit vector perpendicular to the scattering plane. P_l & P_l^1 are regular and associated Legendre polynomials, respectively. The differential cross section for the scattering of the unpolarized incident beam is given by

$$\frac{d\sigma}{d\Omega} = |f|^2 + |g|^2 \qquad \qquad \dots (1.20)$$

and the polarization produced in the unpolarized incident beam due to scattering is given by

$$\boldsymbol{P}(\theta) = \frac{(fg^*+gf^*)}{|f|^2+|g|^2}\,\hat{n} = P(\theta)\hat{n} \qquad \qquad \dots (1.21)$$

where $P(\theta)$ is the Sherman function. Other spin polarization parameters T and U giving the angle of component of the polarization vector in the scattering plane are given by

$$\boldsymbol{T}(\theta) = \frac{|f|^2-|g|^2}{|f|^2+|g|^2} \qquad \qquad \dots (1.22)$$

$$\boldsymbol{U}(\theta) = i\frac{fg^*-gf^*}{|f|^2+|g|^2} \qquad \qquad \dots (1.23)$$

1.2.5 COLLISION STRENGTH AND EFFECTIVE COLLISION STRENGTH

It is convenient to use symmetric and dimensionless collision strength Ω to present result for astrophysical applications than the collision cross section. The collision strength for excitation from level i to level f is related to the cross section σ in units of πa_0^2 by the relation

$$\Omega_{if}(E) = g_i K_i^2 \sigma_{if}(E) \qquad \qquad \dots (1.24)$$

where g_i is the statistical weight of level i and $E = K_i^2$ is the energy in Rydbergs of the incident electron or positron relative to level i. At threshold energy, the collision strength for alkali atom is zero and then it varies with increase of energy depending on the type of transition. In the asymptotic region, the collision strength follows a high energy limiting behaviour. This behaviour is also determined by type of transition. For optically allowed electric dipole transitions, the collision strength is given by relation

$$\Omega_{if}(E)_{E\to\infty} \approx dl_n(E) \qquad\qquad\qquad \text{.... (1.25)}$$

where the parameter d is proportional to the oscillator strength. In the case of multipole optically-forbidden transition such as electric quadrupole or magnetic-dipole transitions, the collision strength is given as

$$\Omega_{if}(E)_{E\to\infty} \approx constant \qquad\qquad\qquad \text{.... (1.26)}$$

In many other astrophysical applications, use of excitation rate coefficients or thermally averaged collision strengths as a function of electron temperature is convenient. The excitation rates are obtained by averaging collision strengths over a Maxwellian distribution of electron energies. The excitation rates coefficient for a transition from state i to f at electron temperature T_e is given by

$$C_{if} = \frac{8.629\times10^{-6}}{g_i T_e^{1/2}} \gamma_{if}(T_e) exp\left(-\frac{\Delta E_{if}}{KT_e}\right) cm^3 S^{-1} \qquad\qquad \text{.... (1.27)}$$

where $g_i = (2J_i + 1)$ is the statistical weight of the lower level i, $\Delta E_{if} = E_f - E_i$ is the excitation energy and γ_{if} is a dimensionless quantity, called effective collision strength, given by

$$\gamma_{if}(T_e) = \int_0^\infty \Omega_{if}\, exp\left(-\frac{E_f}{kT_e}\right) d\left(\frac{E_f}{kT_e}\right) \qquad\qquad \text{.... (1.28)}$$

where E_f is the energy of incident electron or positron with respect to upper level f.

1.3 VARIOUS THEORETICAL APPROXIMATIONS USED IN COLLISION PHYSICS

In quantum mechanical treatment of collision process either time dependent or time independent methods are used. In time independent quantum mechanical approach, it is assumed that incident beam has been acting for a long time so that whole system has reached a stationary state. A collision between an electron and one electron atom (Hydrogen atom) can then be described by the time independent Schrodinger equation

$$(H - E)\psi(\vec{r}_1, \vec{r}_2) = 0 \qquad \qquad \text{.... (1.29)}$$

where $\psi(\vec{r}_1, \vec{r}_2)$ is the wavefunction of entire system *i.e.* incident particle plus target atom. $\vec{r}_1 \& \vec{r}_2$ are the position vectors of the target electron and incident particle respectively. E is the total energy of the system given by

$$E = \frac{\hbar^2 k_i^2}{2\mu} + \epsilon_i = \frac{\hbar^2 k_f^2}{2\mu} + \epsilon_f \qquad \qquad \text{.... (1.30)}$$

$\hbar k_i$ and $\hbar k_f$ are the momenta of incident and scattered particles respectively. μ is the reduced mass of the system. ϵ_i and ϵ_f are the target internal energies in the initial and final channels respectively. In atomic mass unit $\hbar = \mu = e = 1$. H is the total Hamiltonian of the system, given by

$$H = -\frac{\hbar^2}{2\mu}(\nabla_1^2 + \nabla_2^2) - \frac{e^2}{r_1} + V(r_1, r_2) \qquad \qquad \text{.... (1.31)}$$

where $V(r_1, r_2) = \dfrac{Z'e^2}{r_2} - \dfrac{Z'e^2}{|\vec{r_1} - \vec{r_2}|}$ $\qquad \qquad \text{.... (1.32)}$

is the total interaction potential between the incident particle and target, e is the electronic charge and Z' represents the charge on projectile. $\nabla_1^2 \& \nabla_2^2$ are the kinetic energy operators of the atomic electron and incident particle respectively.

For the evaluation of the function $\psi(\vec{r}_1, \vec{r}_2)$ in equation (1.29), various approximation methods have been suggested in the literature depending upon the range of energy in which scattering studies are made. One of the most important methods in quantum theory of scattering from atomic system is eigen function expansion method in which total wave function $\psi(\vec{r}_1, \vec{r}_2)$ of the system is expanded in terms of unperturbed target atom wave function u_n .

$$\psi^{\pm}(\vec{r}_1, \vec{r}_2) = \sum_n [F_n^{\pm}(\vec{r}_2)u_n(\vec{r}_1) \pm F_n^{\pm}(\vec{r}_1)u_n(\vec{r}_2)] \qquad \ldots (1.33)$$

where F_n represents the scattering wavefunction and $\sum_n$ denote the summation over all the discrete states and integration over the continuum states of the target. The plus and minus sign refer to the singlet (symmetric) and triplet (antisymmetric) states respectively. The equation (1.33) can also be written as

$$\psi(\vec{r}_1, \vec{r}_2) = \mathcal{A} \oint_n F_n(\vec{r}_2)u_n(\vec{r}_1) \qquad \ldots\ldots (1.34)$$

Here $\mathcal{A}$ is the antisymmetrization operator which takes into account the exchange effect (in case of electron atom scattering) due to indistinguishability of the projectile and target electron. $\oint$ denotes the summation overall discrete states and integration over the continuum state of the target. We may use either the equations. Combining the equations (1.29) and (1.33) or (1.34), one obtains an infinite set of coupled equations

$$(\nabla^2 + k_n^2)F_n^{\pm}(\vec{r}_2) = \frac{2\mu}{\hbar^2} \sum_m \left[V_{nm}(\vec{r}_2)F_m^{\pm}(\vec{r}_2) \pm \int W_{nm}(\vec{r}_1, \vec{r}_2)F_m^{\pm}(\vec{r}_1)d\vec{r}_1 \right]$$

$$\ldots (1.35)$$

where V_{nm} and W_{nm} are the direct matrix and exchange Kernal operator defined respectively as

$$V_{nm} = \int u_n^*(\vec{r}_1)V(r_1, r_2)u_m(\vec{r}_1)dr_1 \qquad \ldots (1.36)$$

$$W_{nm} = u_n^*(\vec{r}_1)[H - E]u_m(\vec{r}_2) \qquad\qquad \dots (1.37)$$

Asymptotically, the scattering wave function $F(\vec{r}_2)$ can be represented as a superposition of the incident plane wave and an outgoing spherical wave. Therefore

$$F_n^{\pm}(\vec{r}_2)_{r_2 \to \infty} \approx \exp(i\vec{k}_n.r_2)\delta n_i + \frac{1}{r_2} f_n^{\pm}(\theta, \phi)\exp(ik_n r_2) \qquad\qquad \dots (1.38)$$

where $f_n^{\pm}(\theta, \phi)$ is the direct inelastic scattering amplitude for the transition in which the incident electron is scattered and the atomic electron is excited to some another level. The complete set of coupled integro-differential equation (1.35) is practically solvable and so one requires an approximation to solve them. In general the differential scattering cross section is defined as

$$\frac{d\sigma}{d\Omega} = \frac{k_n}{k_i}\left[\frac{1}{4}|f_n^+(\theta, \phi)|^2 + \frac{3}{4}|f_n^-(\theta, \phi)|^2\right] \qquad\qquad \dots (1.39)$$

For elastic scattering $n = 1$.

Let us now discuss few important theoretical approximations commonly used in various collision processes.

1.3.1 FIRST BORN APPROXIMATION

In quantum mechanical treatment of scattering theory, if the scattering potential is weak such that scattering does not take place at a large distance then Born approximation can be used to evaluate the scattering amplitude $f(\theta, \phi)$ and hence the differential cross section $\sigma(\theta, \phi) = |f(\theta, \phi)|^2$. Considering the mass of nucleus which is more than the mass of electron and taking it as origin, the whole system can be explained by the time independent non relativistic Schrodinger equation

$$H\psi(\vec{r}_1, \vec{r}_2) = E\psi(\vec{r}_1, \vec{r}_2) \qquad\qquad \dots (1.40)$$

Here $\psi(\vec{r}_1, \vec{r}_2)$ is the total wave function. $\vec{r}_1$ & $\vec{r}_2$ are the position coordinates of the target and incident particle respectively. H is the total Hamiltonian of the system (incident plus target) given as

$$H = -\frac{\hbar^2}{2\mu}\, \nabla_2^2 + H_A(r_1) + V(r_1, r_2) \qquad \ldots\ (1.41)$$

Here H_A is the Hamiltonian of target (one electron atom) given by

$$H_A = -\frac{\hbar^2}{2\mu}\, \nabla_1^2 - \frac{e^2}{r_1} \qquad \ldots\ (1.42)$$

And total interaction potential between the incident particle and target atom is

$$V(\vec{r}_1, \vec{r}_2) = \frac{Z\,Z'\,e^2}{|\vec{r}_2|} - \frac{Z'\,e^2}{|\vec{r}_1 - \vec{r}_2|} \qquad \ldots\ (1.43)$$

Where e is the electronic charge, Z' be the charge on projectile, Z is the atomic number of target. ∇_1^2 & ∇_2^2 are the kinetic energy operators of atomic electron and incident particle respectively.

In equation (1.40), there are so many methods to obtain the wave function $\psi(\vec{r}_1, \vec{r}_2)$. In eigen function expansion method for the investigation and analysis of electron (positron) atom scattering, the total wave function is expanded in term of complete specified state of unperturbed target wave function V_n.

$$\psi(\vec{r}_1, \vec{r}_2) = \mathcal{A} \int \Sigma\, F_n(\vec{r}_2) V_n(\vec{r}_1) \qquad \ldots\ (1.44)$$

In case of electron-atom scattering, antisymmetrization operator ($\mathcal{A}$) takes a description of exchange effect caused by the inability to identified projectile and target electron. F_n is the scattered particle wave function and represent the process of adding all discrete states and integrating over the continuum states of the target equation (1.40) and (1.44). Then finite group of coupled equations can be obtained.

$$(\nabla_2^2 + K_n^2)\, F_n^\pm(\vec{r}_2) = \frac{2\mu}{\hbar^2} \sum_m \left[V_{nm}(\vec{r}_2) F_m^\pm(\vec{r}_2) \pm \int W_{nm}(\vec{r}_1,\vec{r}_2) F^\pm(\vec{r}_1)\,d\vec{r}_1 \right]$$

$$\dots (1.45)$$

Here $\pm$ sign shows singlet and triplet spin states respectively. The direct matrix and exchange kernel operators are represented by V_{nm} and W_{nm} respectively as follows.

$$\left.\begin{aligned} V_{nm} &= \int V_n^*(\vec{r}_1) V(\vec{r}_1,\vec{r}_2) V_m(\vec{r}_1)\,d\vec{r}_1 \\ W_{nm} &= V_n^*(\vec{r}_1)\,(H - E) V_m(\vec{r}_2) \end{aligned}\right\} \qquad \dots (1.46)$$

By the superposition of incident plane wave and outgoing spherical wave, scattering wave function can be obtained

$$F_n^\pm(\vec{r}_2)_{n\to\infty} \sim e^{i(\vec{K}_n.\vec{r}_2)}\,\delta_{ni} + \frac{1}{r_2} f_{in}^\pm(\theta,\phi)\, e^{iK_n r_2} \qquad \dots (1.47)$$

$f_{in}^\pm(\theta,\phi)$ is associated with scattering amplitude for transition of target atom from initial state i to some state n.

The correct solution of equation (1.45) in term of an inhomogeneous integral equation can be written as

$$\begin{aligned} F_n^\pm(\vec{r}_2) \;=\; & \exp(ik_i.r_2)\delta_{ni} + \frac{2\mu}{\hbar^2}\int G_m(\vec{r}_2,\vec{r}_2')\, V_{nm}(\vec{r}_2') F_m(\vec{r}_2')\,d\vec{r}_2' \;+ \\[4pt] & \frac{2\mu}{\hbar^2}\int G_m(\vec{r}_2,\vec{r}_2')\, W_{nm}(\vec{r}_2,\vec{r}_1) F_m(\vec{r}_1)\,d\vec{r}_2'\,d\vec{r}_1 \qquad \dots (1.48a) \end{aligned}$$

Here $G_m(\vec{r}_2,\vec{r}_2')$ represents Green function and is given by

$$G_m(\vec{r}_2,\vec{r}_2') = -\frac{1}{4\pi}\exp\frac{(ik_m|\vec{r}_2-\vec{r}_2'|)}{|\vec{r}_2-\vec{r}_2'|} \qquad \dots (1.48b)$$

Adopting the asymptotic form of Green function in above equation and describing the resemblance of it with equation (1.47), we move into a specified position as follows

$$f_n^\pm(\vec{k}_n,\vec{k}_i) = f_{in}(\vec{k}_n,\vec{k}_i) \pm g_{in}(\vec{k}_n,\vec{k}_i) \qquad \dots (1.49)$$

Accepting the responsibility, in which $f_{in}\left(\vec{k}_n,\vec{k}_i\right)$ and $g_{in}\left(\vec{k}_n,\vec{k}_i\right)$ are the direct and exchange scattering amplitudes respectively given by

$$f_{in}\left(\vec{k}_n,\vec{k}_i\right) = -\frac{1}{2\pi}\frac{\mu}{\hbar^2}\int \exp(-ik_n.\vec{r}_2')V_{nm}(\vec{r}_2')F_m(\vec{r}_2')d\vec{r}_2' \qquad \text{..... (1.50a)}$$

$$g_{in}\left(\vec{k}_n,\vec{k}_i\right) = -\frac{1}{2\pi}\frac{\mu}{\hbar^2}\int \exp(-ik_n.\vec{r}_2')W_{nm}(\vec{r}_2',\vec{r}_1)F_m(\vec{r}_1)d\vec{r}_2'dr_1 \qquad \text{.... (1.50b)}$$

Born series, in favour of scattering amplitudes f_{in} and g_{in}, can be achieved by integrating the solution of above said equation. The approximation methods will be genuine tool to solve exact solution of these integral equations.

Taking into account the first Born (FB) approximation, we think carefully about perturbation to be very weak and similarly projectile wave function can be denoted by simple plane wave. By retaining only the first leading term in the series expansion and neglecting exchange, the first Born term can be obtained. So that scattering amplitude taking into account as follows.

$$\left.\begin{array}{l} F_{B_1} = \frac{1}{2\pi}\frac{\mu}{\hbar^2}\int \exp(i\vec{q}.\vec{r}_2)V_{fi}(\vec{r}_2)d\vec{r}_2 \\[2mm] V_{fi} = \langle V_f|V|V_i\rangle \end{array}\right\} \qquad \text{.... (1.51)}$$

The momentum transfer during collision is $\vec{q} = \left(\vec{k}_i - \vec{k}_f\right)$. The authenticity of this approximation can be expected both at very high energy and at small momentum transfer q.

1.3.2 SECOND BORN APPROXIMATION

The FBA which is suitable for high energies completely neglects the effects due to the polarization of target by incident electron and the distortion of the incident plane wave. These effects become important as the incident energy is lowered. The second Born approximation (SBA) takes into account the distortion of the target. The scattering amplitude in this approximation can be written as

$$F_{B2} = F_{fi}^{(1)} + F_{fi}^{(2)} \qquad\qquad \text{.... (1.52)}$$

where $f_{fi}^{(2)}$ is the second-Born scattering amplitude given by the equation

$$F_{fi}^{(2)} = -\frac{1}{\pi}\frac{\mu^2}{\hbar^4}\sum_m \int exp\{i(\vec{k}_i.\vec{r}_2' - \vec{k}_f.\vec{r}_2)\}G_m(\vec{r}_2,\vec{r}_2')V_{fm}(\vec{r}_2)V_{mi}(\vec{r}_2')d\vec{r}_2 d\vec{r}_2'$$

$$\text{.... (1.53)}$$

This approximation involves a summation over infinite number of intermediate states. This may be done by assuming the target excited states to be completely degenerate with its ground state *i.e.* the energy of the intermediate state is taken to be fixed and is equal the ground state energy itself. The summation is taken easily done by the closure property. Holt and Moisewitsch [14] and Holt *et al* [15] have considered the first few target states explicitly and the effects of the rest is included by replacing the energies of the intermediate state by an average excitation energy.

The FBA fails as the strength of the potential increases. Therefore one has to consider higher Born terms in the born series, which are rather difficult to evaluate. Some high energy semi classical approximations such as the Eikonal and Glauber have been widely used in the study of the scattering of electrons by atomic targets.

1.3.3 BORN-HARTREE-BETHE APPROXIMATION

Born-Hartree-Bethe approximation is a new method in the theory of high energy electron-atom/molecule scattering taking account the completeness property of atomic and molecular wavefunctions in the framework of first Born approximation. The main advantage of this approximation is that the total integral cross section (TICS) can be calculated by minimum available information on the target namely its ground state wavefunction and mean excitation energy; no other parameters or assumptions are needed. In the first Born approximation, when electron with initial momentum P, scatters on the many electron target (atom or molecule), the transition probability from the initial state $|i\rangle$ with energy E_i to the final state $|f\rangle$ with energy E_f is determined by

$$dw_{i\to f} = 2\pi |\langle fP'|U|iP\rangle|^2 \delta\left(\frac{P'^2-P^2}{2} + E_f - E_i\right)\frac{dp'}{(2\pi)^3} \qquad \dots (1.54)$$

where $\quad U = \sum_{j=1}^{A}\frac{Z_i}{|r-R_j|} - \sum_{j=1}^{N}\frac{1}{|r-r_j|}$ $\qquad \dots (1.55)$

is the interaction potential of the incident electron and the atom composed of a nuclei with charges Z_j, coordinates R_j and N electrons.

The differential cross section (DCS) of electron scattering for the transition from molecular state $|i\rangle$ to state $|f\rangle$ is

$$\frac{d\sigma_{i\to f}}{d\Omega} = \frac{p'}{4\pi^2 p}\left|\int\langle f|U\,e^{-iqr}|i\rangle dr\right|^2 \qquad \dots (1.56)$$

where $q = p - p'$ is the electron momentum transfer.

1.3.4 MODIFIED BORN APPROXIMATION(MB)

The Born approximation was modified by Junker [16]. The total Hamiltonian for the system (projectile plus target atom) may be written as

$$H = H_0 + V \qquad \dots (1.57)$$

where H_0 is the unperturbed part of is total Hamiltonian and V is the total interaction potential between the colliding particle and target atom. It can be divided as

$$H = H_0 + U + W$$

or $\qquad H = H_1 + W$ $\qquad \dots (1.58)$

with $\quad H_1 = H_0 + U$

where $U = \dfrac{z'\delta}{r_{N+1}}$

and $W = \dfrac{z'(Z-\delta)}{r_{N+1}} - \sum_{i=1}^{N} \dfrac{z'}{r_{iN+1}}$

Z is the total nuclear charge and δ is the screening parameter.

The Schrodinger equation with Hamiltonian H_0, H_1 and H respectively given by

$$\left.\begin{array}{l} H_0\phi_r = E\phi_r \\ H_1\chi_r = E\chi_r \\ H\psi_r = E\psi_r \end{array}\right\} \qquad \dots (1.59)$$

The T-matrix element for a collision from initial state i to final state f is given by

$$T_{i\to f} = \langle \phi_f|V|\psi_i^+\rangle \qquad \dots (1.60)$$

The function ψ_i^+ satisfying the outgoing boundary conditions can be expressed with respect to H_1.

$$\psi_i^+ = \sum_{n=0}^{\infty}\left(G^{(+)}W\right)^n \chi_i^{(+)} \qquad \dots (1.61)$$

Where G^+ is the Green function for the Hamiltonian H_1 . This corresponds to expanding ψ_i^+ in a series about an effective number charge δ instead of zero. Retaining only the first term one obtains

$$T_{i\to f}^{MB} = \langle \phi_f|V|\chi_i^{(+)}\rangle \qquad \dots (1.62)$$

1.3.5 COULOMB BORN APPROXIMATION (CB)

This approximation is useful in describing collision of electrons (positrons) and ions with target ions, in which the Coulomb interaction of projectile with the target can be important. The Born plane wave functions are replaced by Coulomb wave functions corresponding to nuclear charge. For highly charged ions, the long range Coulomb interaction becomes dominant, and all other interaction can be treated as small perturbations. The Coulomb Born approximation (CBA) is never good for electron-neutral atoms scattering. One of the special classes of the distorted wave approximation was proposed by Geltman [17] and Geltman and Hidalgo [18]. In this approach the total Hamiltonian of the system (projectile plus target atom) is partitioned as

$$H = H_0^{'} + V^{'} \qquad \qquad \dots (1.63)$$

where $H_0^{'}$ is the unperturbed Hamiltonian which includes the projectile-target nucleus interaction, and $V^{'}$ contains the projectile interaction with the target electrons i.e.

$$V^{'} = -\sum_{i=1}^{n} \frac{Z^{'}}{r_{iN+1}} \qquad \qquad \dots (1.64)$$

where N is the number of electrons in the target atoms, $\vec{r}_{N+1}$ and $\vec{r}_i$ are the position coordinates of the incident particle and the target electrons respectively. $Z^{'}$ is equal to -1 for electron and +1 for positron or proton.

The T-matrix element for a collision in which the target atom is excited from initial state 'i' to final state 'f' is given by

$$T_{i \to f} = \langle \chi_f^{(-)} | V^{'} | \Psi_i^{(+)} \rangle \qquad \qquad \dots (1.65)$$

Here $\Psi_i^{(+)}$ is the solution of Schrodinger's equation

$$(H - E)\Psi_i^{(+)} = 0 \qquad \qquad \dots (1.66)$$

which satisfy the outgoing boundary condition, denoted by the superscript. E is the total energy of the system.

With the choice of splitting considered by Geltman and Hidalgo [19] the Hamiltonian H_0' remains a separate Hamiltonian for which one can obtain the exact Eigen function $\chi_f^{(-)}$

$$(H - E)\chi_f^{(-)} = 0 \qquad\qquad \ldots (1.67)$$

Making the first Born approximation for $\Psi_i^{(+)}$, Geltman and Hidalgo [19] obtain

$$T_{i\to f}^{CB} = \langle \chi_f^{(-)}|V'|\phi_i\rangle \qquad\qquad \ldots (1.68)$$

1.3.6 DISTORTED WAVE BORN APPROXIMATION (DWBA)

Suppose we have an electron with momentum k_i which collide with an atom A, after the collision, the scattered electron has the momentum k_f , and one bound electron in atom A is excited to higher energy bound state. In the frozen core approximation, the exact Hamiltonian for the whole system is

$$H = -\frac{1}{2}\nabla_1^2 + V_{A^+}(\vec{r}_1) - \frac{1}{2}\nabla_2^2 + V_{A^+}(\vec{r}_2) + \frac{1}{r_{12}} \qquad \ldots (1.69)$$

Where $\vec{r}_1$ and $\vec{r}_2$ are position vectors for the projectile and the bound state electron with respect to the nucleus respectively. This Hamiltonian can be rewritten approximately as

$$H_j = -\frac{1}{2}\nabla_1^2 + U_j(r_1) - \frac{1}{2}\nabla_2^2 + V_{A^+}(r_2) \quad (j = i, f) \qquad \ldots (1.70)$$

In this equation $U_i\left(U_f\right)$ is the distorting potential used to calculate the initial (final) state wavefunction χ_{k_i} (χ_{k_f}) for the projectile. In the DWBA, the direct transition amplitude for excitation from an initial state Ψ_i to a final state Ψ_f is expressed by

$$f = \langle \chi_{k_f}^{-}(1)\Psi_f(2)|V_i|\Psi_i(2)\,\chi_{k_i}^{+}(1)\rangle \qquad\qquad \ldots (1.71)$$

where V_i is the perturbation interaction:

$$V_i = H - H_i = \frac{1}{r_{12}} + V_{A^+}(r_1) - U_i(r_1) \qquad \text{.... (1.72)}$$

In equation (1.71), the initial and final state wave functions for the projectile satisfy the differential equation

$$\left[-\frac{1}{2}\nabla_1^2 + U_j(r_1) - \frac{1}{2}k_j^2\right]\chi_{k_j}(r_1) = 0 \qquad (j = i,f) \qquad \text{.... (1.73)}$$

and the bound state wave functions are the eigen functions of the equation

$$\left[-\frac{1}{2}\nabla_2^2 + V_{A^+}(r_2) - \epsilon_j\right]\Psi_j(r_2) = 0 \qquad (j = i,f) \qquad \text{.... (1.74)}$$

where ϵ_j $(j = i,f)$ are the corresponding eigenergies of the initial and final bound states which can be expressed as

$$\Psi_j(\vec{r}) = \Psi_{N_j L_j}(r)\, Y_{L_j M_j}(\hat{r}) \qquad (j = i,f) \qquad \text{.... (1.75)}$$

The exchange scattering amplitude is given by

$$g = \langle \Psi_f(1)\chi_{k_f}^-(2)|V_i|\Psi_i(2)\,\chi_{k_i}^+(1)\rangle \qquad \text{.... (1.76)}$$

Finally, the differential cross section for electron impact excitation is given by

$$\frac{d\sigma}{d\Omega} = N(2\pi)^4\frac{k_f}{k_i}\frac{1}{2L_i+1} \times \sum_{M_i=-L_i}^{+L_i}\sum_{M_f=-L_f}^{+L_f}\left(\frac{3}{4}|f-g|^2 + \frac{1}{4}|f+g|^2\right) \qquad \text{.... (1.77)}$$

The prefactor N in equation (1.77) denotes the number of electrons in the sub shell from which one electron is excited.

The distorting potentials U_i and U_f, used in equation (1.73) to calculate the wavefunctions for the projectile in the initial and final states, respectively, are not determined directly by the formalism. Here, we use static potential which take the form as

$$U_j(r_1) = V_{A^+}(r_1) + \int dr_2 \frac{|\Psi_j(r_2)|^2}{r_{12}} \qquad (j = i, f) \qquad \dots (1.78)$$

As shown previously, $V_{A^+}(r)$ in equation (1.78) is the atomic potential used to evaluate eigenstate wavefunctions of the bound state electron. Here we use the effective potential from Tong and Lin [19] based on single active electron approximation, which is given by

$$V_{A^+}(r) = -\frac{1 + a_1 e^{-a_2 r} + a_3 r\, e^{-a_4 r} + a_5 e^{-a_6 r}}{r} \qquad \dots (1.79)$$

where the parameters a_i are obtained by fitting the calculated binding energies from the potential to experimental ones of the ground state and the first few excited states of the target atom.

1.3.7   CLOSE COUPLING APPROXIMATION

Now we shall start to deal with in a certain way that provides us to get a crystal clear concept of all physical aspects of scattering problem. Basically, it consists of an expansion of total wave function in term of eigen function of the bound sub systems with unknown scattering coefficient. These unknown expansion coefficients are then determined as the solution of a set of coupled integro-differential equations whose number will depend on the number of eigen states included in the expansion. Generally, in practice, few lowest lying states are included giving rise to a finite set of coupled equations. The problem with this method lies infact that any appropriate basis set must contain a major contribution from the continuous states which either be ignored or treated in some approximate manner. In close coupling approximation such expansion is converged after retaining the first few atomic states. If the eigen function retained are labeled from $m = 1$ to $m = N$, the system of N coupled equations is written as

$$(\nabla_2^2 + K_n^2)F_n^{\pm}(\vec{r}_2) = \frac{2\mu}{\hbar^2}\sum_{m=1}^{N}[V_{nm}\,F_n^{\pm}(\vec{r}_2) \pm \int W_{nm}\,(\vec{r}_1,\vec{r}_2)F_n^{\pm}(\vec{r}_1)d\vec{r}_1] \qquad .... (1.80)$$

1.3.8 EIKONAL APPROXIMATION

When wavelength of the projectile is small compared with the distance over which the scattering potential changes appreciably, the concept of classical trajectory acquires meaning. If r_0 is the change in the potential, the condition may be stated as

$$k\,r_0 \gg 1 \qquad\qquad .... (1.81)$$

This condition is the basis of semi classical scattering approximations, which have been very useful for heavy particle, and also for electron scattering. Further, if the energy of the projectile, E, is large compared with a typical value of potential, V_0, so that

$$\frac{V_0}{E} \ll 1 \qquad\qquad .... (1.82)$$

The eikonal approach to the scattering problems becomes feasible, as we shall show here. First let us consider the classical limit of time independent wave equation for the projectile-target relative motion in classical scattering by a structureless potential V(r)

$$\left[-\frac{\hbar^2}{2m} + V(r) - E\right]\Psi(r) = 0 \qquad\qquad .... (1.83)$$

We write

$$\Psi(r) = e^{\frac{iS(r)}{\hbar}} \qquad\qquad .... (1.84)$$

and obtain

$$\frac{1}{2m}[-i\hbar\nabla^2 S + (\nabla S)^2] = E - V(r) \qquad \text{.... (1.85)}$$

We go to classical limit when $\nabla^2 S \ll (\nabla S)^2$, this condition being equivalent to the limit. In this limit, $S = S_0(r)$, and

$$\frac{1}{2m}(\nabla S_0)^2 = E - V(r) \qquad \text{.... (1.86)}$$

If $S_0(r)$ is taken to be Hamiltonian's characteristic function, is the classical Hamiltonian-Jacobi equation. In optics this equation is called the eikonal equation. By integrating, we can determine the trajectories that are normal to the surface $S_0(r)$ = constant. Since normal to the surface are parallel to ∇S, formal solution of equation (1.86) is

$$S_0(r) = \int ds \{2m\,|E - V(r)|\} \qquad \text{.... (1.87)}$$

where the integration is along a trajectory. If we substitute S into (1.84), we obtain the eikonal wave function. The use of this approximate wave function in the integral equation for the scattering amplitude is basis of the eikonal approximation. This approximation is most accurate for high impact energies or for weak interactions. It represents the relative motion of the collision partners by a distorted plane wave, and may be regarded as first order correction to the Born approximation, which treats the relative motion as an undistorted plane wave. If the impact energy greatly exceeds the interaction energy and the internal energy of the system, the trajectory of the system will not deviate significantly from a straight line path.

1.3.9 R-MATRIX THEORY

The R-matrix theory introduced by Wigner and Eisenbud in 1947, is a powerful nuclear interaction model. It is a well established ab-initio formalism to calculate differential, integral and momentum-transfer cross sections for elastic scattering of electron by molecule. In R-matrix approach [20,21], the configuration space of scattering system is divided into two spatial regions; an inner region and an outer region. These regions are treated differently in accordance with the different interactions in each region. The centre if R-matrix sphere coincides with the centre of molecule. When the scattering electron leaves the inner region, the outer target electrons are confined to the inner region. The R-matrix boundary radius dividing the two regions is taken to be $n\,a_0$ centred at the molecular centre of mass. This sphere encloses entire charge cloud of the occupied and virtual molecular orbitals included in the calculation. However, the continuum orbitals have finite amplitudes at the boundary inside the R-matrix sphere, the electron-electron correlation and exchange interactions are strong. Short range correlation effects are important for accurate prediction of large angle elastic scattering. A multi-centered configuration interaction wave function expansion is used in the inner region. The calculation in the inner region is similar to the bound state calculation, which involves the solution of an eigen value problem for (N+1) electrons in the truncated space, where there are N target electrons and a single scattering electron. Most of the physics of the scattering problem is contained in this (N+1) electrons bound state molecular structure calculation. Outside the sphere, only long-range multi-polar interactions between the scattering electron and the various target states are included. Since only direct potentials are involved in the outer region, a single centre approach is used to describe the scattering electron via a set of coupled differential equations. The R-matrix is a mathematical entity that connects the two regions. It describes how the scattering electron enters the inner region and how it leaves it. In the outer region, the R-matrix on the boundary is propagated outwards [22,23] until the inner region solutions can be matched with asymptotic solutions thus yielding the physical observables like cross sections. We include only the dipole and quadruple moments in the outer region.

In the polyatomic implementation of the R-matrix code [24,25], the continuum molecular orbitals are constructed from atomic Gaussian type orbitals (GTOs) using basis functions centered on the centre of gravity of the molecule. The main advantage of GTOs is that integrals involving them over all space can be evaluated analytically in closed form. However, a tail contribution is subtracted to yield the required integral in the truncated space defined by inner region [24].

The target molecular orbital space is divided into core (inactive), valence (active) and virtual orbitals. The target molecular orbitals are supplemented with a set of continuum orbitals, centered on the centre of gravity of the molecule. The continuum basis functions used in polyatomic R-matrix calculations are Gaussian functions and do not require fixed boundary conditions. First, target and continuum molecular orbitals are orthogonalized using Schmidt orthonalization. Then symmetric or Lowdin orthonalization is used to orthogonalize the continuum molecular orbitals among themselves and remove linearly dependent functions [24,26]. In general all the calculations are performed within the fixed-nuclei approximation. This is based on the assumption in which electronic, vibrational and rotational motions are uncoupled.

In inner region, the wave function of the scattering system consisting of target plus scattering electron is written using the configuration interaction expression:

$$\Psi_k^{N+1} = A \sum_i \phi_i^N(X_1, \dots X_N) \sum_j \xi_i(X_{N+1}) a_{ijk} + \sum_m \chi_m(X_1, \dots X_N, X_{N+1}) b_{mk}$$

$$\dots (1.88)$$

Where, A is an anti-symmetrization operator, X_N is the spatial and spin coordinate of Nth electron, ϕ_i^N represents the ith state of N-electron target, ξ_i is a continuum orbital spin coupled with the scattering electron, k refers to a particular R-matrix basis function. Coefficients a_{ijk} and b_{mk} are vibrational parameters determined as a result of matrix diagonalization. To obtain reliable results, it is important to maintain balance between the N-electron target representation, ϕ_i^N, and the (N+1) electron scattering wave function. The summation in the second term of equation (1.88) runs over configurations χ_m, where all electrons placed in target occupied and virtual molecular orbitals. The choice of appropriate χ_m is crucial [27]. These are known as L^2 configurations and are needed, to account for orthogonality relaxation and for correlation effects arising from virtual excitation to higher electronic state that are excluded in the first expansion. The basis for continuum electron is parametrically dependent on the R-matrix radius and provides a good approximation to an equivalent basis of orthonormal spherical Bessel functions [28].

1.3.10 THEORETICAL SURVEY OF APPROXIMATION METHODS

We have done exhaustive theoretical and experimental survey of literature. But here we are mentioning a few of them.

Chen and Msezane [29] have been studied correlation effects in the generalized oscillator strength of Magnesium 3^1S-3^1P transition by comparing the results calculated within the random phase approximation by Hartee-Fock calculations. The polarization alignment and orientation studies in Cesium atom have presented by Anderson and Bartschat [30]. Chen *et al* [31] have calculated electron impact excitation of Iron using Breit-Pauli R-matrix theory. The close coupling method have been illustrated by Bartschat *et al* [32] at low energy electron scattering from Magnesium. The electron impact coherence parameters for excitation in Barium have been calculated by Muktawat *et al* [33]. Predojevic *et al* [34] have measured the differential cross section for electron impact excitation of resonance state of Ytterbium. Elastic to inelastic intensity ratio are also obtained from energy loss spectra record. Berrington *et al* [35] have also found the collision strength and excitation rates for electron impact on ionized Iron element using Dirac R-matrix method. An eikonal model for electron excitation and loss from highly charged ionic projectiles colliding with atomic targets at relativistic collision energies is given by Voitkiv [36], in which distortion of the target transition by the strong field of the projectile nucleus is taken into account using the symmetric eikonal approximation. General expressions are derived for the eikonal transition amplitude in the case of collisions with one and two-electron targets. By discussing the relativistic features and nonrelativistic limit of the eikonal transition amplitude he has shown that the higher-order terms in the projectile-target interaction, which are not accounted for by the first-order amplitude, may be of importance even for quite small values of Z p (the charge of the projectile nucleus) and v (the collision velocity). Srivastava *et al* [37] have used relativistic distorted wave approximation to calculate the lowest metastable state of neon, argon, krypton and xenon to the ten higher lying fine structure levels of the $n\,p^5(n+1)p$ configuration. Christopher and Zhang [38] have presented an exact treatment of the relativistic plane-wave Born (RPWB) cross section for electron impact excitation for an arbitrary atom and ion. This result represents an improvement over the cross section obtained from the widely used Bethe high-energy theory. The results obtained from this RPWB approach can be applied to a broad class of problems in fundamental electron-impact scattering theory. Y. Ishikawa [49] has used relativistic R-matrix close-coupling method based on effective many-body Hamiltonians to calculate the electron-impact excitations of intercombination transitions in the Kr6+ ion. Badnell [40] have described the development of the Dirac R-matrix with pseudo-states (DRMPS) method for electron and photon collisions with arbitrary atoms and ions. Very recently Rajvanshi and Baluja [41] presented elastic integrated and differential cross section (DCS), momentum transfer, excitation, and ionization cross sections for electron impact on S_2 molecules using R-matrix method.

1.4 RECENT EXPERIMENTAL WORK IN PRESENT SCENARIO

The comparisons of experiments with available results serve the purpose of illustrating the success, authenticity and limitations of the particular method over the other. Using method of gas mixtures, Khakoo *et al* [42] have reported electron-impact differential cross section measurements for excitation of the $2p^53s$ configuration of Neon using experimental cross section for electron-impact excitation of $n = 2$ levels of atomic Hydrogen. Ariyasinghe and Goains [43] reported total electron scattering cross sections for Krypton and Xenon for 250–4500 eV electrons by measurement of the electron-beam intensity attenuation through a gas cell. These cross sections are compared with the previous experimental measurements and the predictions by theoretical and semi-empirical models. The discrepancies in experimental cross sections between different experimental groups are explained using the oscillator strengths and inelastic threshold of electron-energy-loss spectra. The correlation between the total electron scattering cross section and the atomic radius is discussed for Neon, Argon, Krypton, and Xenon atoms. Allan [44] has been measured absolute angle-differential cross sections for electron impact excitation of Argon and Xenon atoms to the lowest four $np^5(n + 1)S$ levels and the $5p^5 5d[7/2]_3$ respectively as a function of electron energy upto a few eV above threshold at a fixed scattering angle of 135^0. For Argon very good agreement is observed between their experimental data and predictions from a Breit-Pauli B-spline R-matrix (BSR) method. Stevenson and Lohmann [45] measured the triple differential cross section for electron impact ionization of the 3p orbital of Argon by 113.5 eV incident electrons using a magnetic angle chamber in a conventional (e,2e) spectrometer. The results are presented for 2 eV ejected electrons over an extended angular range and over the complete coplanar scattering plane for 5 eV ejected electrons. Using crossed beam apparatus, Hashino *et al* [46] presented experimental differential cross section for electron impact excitation of $n = 2$ states in Helium. Their measured data is in very good accord with convergent close coupling approach. Caradonna *et al* [47] have been used high resolution ($\Delta E \sim 55meV$) trap-based positron beam to measure absolute scattering cross section for the excitation of resolved 2^1S states of Helium at energies between threshold and 38 eV. Lukasz Klosowski *et al* [48] have measured electron impact coherence parameters for inelastic electron Helium scattering for the excitation to the $2\,^1$P1 state at collision energy of 100 eV. The experiment is conducted using angular correlation electron photon coincidence technique with a magnetic angle changer allowing measurements in full range of scattering angles. The results are compared with other experimental data and theoretical predictions available for this collisional system. Stevenson *et al* [49] have been measured differential cross section for electron-impact ionization of Neon and Xenon describing the post collision interactions. They performed experiment under coplanar asymmetric kinematics, at intermediate incident electron energies, and for a range of scattered electron detection angles. The differential cross sections (DCS) for inelastic electron scattering to the $n = 2$ states in Helium have been measured at incident energies of 80, 100 and 120 eV by Ward *et al* [50] across the complete angular scattering range $(0–180^0)$ using a magnetic angle changer (MAC) with a soft-iron core. The convergent close-coupling (CCC), R-matrix with pseudo states (RMPS), and B-spline R-matrix (BSR) methods have been used to calculate these DCS. An agreement between the experimental data and the predictions from these highly sophisticated theoretical methods is generally good. Jones *et al* [51] have performed high resolution measurements of positron interactions with Neon and Argon over a range of energy 0.3 to 60 eV and comparise measurements of grand total, positronium formation and grand total minus positron formation cross sections. The measurements are performed using a "Surko" buffer-gas trap and beam apparatus. Very recently Zecca *et al* [52] have developed the Trento University spectrometer in which they used a Tungsten moderator of thickness 1micrometer in conjunction with Sodium isotopes as a radiative and some electrostatic optics in order to produce the positron beam. They measured positron Argon total cross section which has good agreement with corresponding available data except lowest energies of common measurement. Excellent qualitative agreement is also found between their measurements and improved convergent close coupling (CCC) calculation.

1.5 BROAD OUTLINES OF PRESENT THESIS WORK

The authors aim to present thesis is to explore new insight in to field of scattering and investigation of scattering of charged particles ($e^{\pm}$) by rare gases as atomic target. The subject matter is based on various suitable quantum mechanical approaches. To regulate the endeavor, firstly a comparative study is made for several excited state of Helium from ground state at various energies of projectile electrons within the framework of pseudo state close-coupling approximation. In this method we have taken a frozen core approximation *i.e.* first electron of target is taken into lowest orbit while second electron is described by a set of non orthogonal of Laguerre-L^2 basis function for 2^1S and 3^1S excited state of Helium. In third chapter we extend our work to the elastic and inelastic scattering of Neon atom by electron impact at numerous energies. In calculation of elastic scattering differential cross section (DCS) which is outcome of solutions of radial Dirac equations, the exchange between the projectile and atomic electrons is accounted by adding a local correction to the traditional electrostatic interaction potential in the view of Buhring's power series method based on cubic-spline interpolation. In determination of inelastic DCS, we consider distorted wave Born approximation in which bound state electron wavefunction is determined by taking some parameters calculated by Tom and Lin [53]. In fourth chapter, we have extended our work broaden till the elastic scattering of Argon by electron as well as positron at numerous impact energies. In calculation of DCS by solving the Dirac equation, we use a model potential to represent the interactions between the positrons and electrons and Argon atom. For each impact energy, the phase shifts of lower partial waves are obtained exactly by numerical integration of radial wave equation. The Born approximation is used to obtain contribution of higher partial waves to the scattering amplitude. In addition, integrated elastic cross section is studied also. 4s and 4p excited state of Argon by electron impact is studied at different impact energies. In inelastic scattering we adopt Born-Hartree-Bethe approximation taking the completeness property of atomic wavefunction. Calculation of TICS under the frame work of first Born approximation, involves only ground state wavefunction and requires no adjustment parameter. In fifth chapter we have calculated differential and total scattering cross section of 5s [3/2] and 5s[1/2] excitation states of Krypton at low projectile energies of electron using the Hartree-Fock wavefunctions. The last chapter presents the summary along with application and future aspect of present work.

<u>REFERENCES</u>

1.   J. B. Boffard, C. C. Lin, C. A. DeJoseph, J. Phys. D **37**, R143 (2004).

2.   A. Hartgers, J. van Dijk, J. Jonkers and J.A.M. van der Mullen, Computt. Phys. Commun.**135**, 199(2001).

3.   R .L .Wahl, *Principles and Practice of Positron Emission Tomography* (Philadelphia, PA: Lippincott Williams and Wilkins) ,(2002).

4.   P. J. Schultz and K. G. Lynn, Rev. *Mod. Phys.* **60,** 701(1988).

5.   See articles Xu J and Moxom J (ed) Proc. 7th Int. Conf. on Positron and Positron Chemistry, Radiation Physics and Chemistry vol. **68** (Amsterdam: Pergamon) pp 329–680(2003).

6.   C. M. Surko, M. Leventhal, W. S. Crane, A .Passner and F .Wysocki, *Rev. Sci. Instrum.* **57** ,1862(1986).

7.   C. M. Surko and R. G. Greaves, *Phys. Plasmas* **11,** 2333(2004).

8.   L. D. Hulett, D. L. Donohue, J. Xu, T. A .Lewis, S .A .McLuckey and G. L. Glish, *Chem. Phys. Lett.* **216,** 236(1993).

9.   U. Fano and J. Macek, Rev. Mod. Phys. **45,** 553 (1973).

10.   L. A. Morgan and M. R. C. McDowell, J. Phys. B**8,** 1073 (1975).

11.   M. Eminyan, K. MacAdam, J. Slevin and H. Kleinpopen, J. Phys.**B7,** 1519 (1974).

12.   N. Sultana, Nahar and J. M. Wadehra, Phys. Rev. A **35**, 2051(1987).

13. C. J. Joachain, Quantum Collision theory (North-Holland, Amsterdam, 1983) Chapt.18.

14. A. R. Holt and B. L. Moisewitsch, J. Phys. **B1**, 36-47(1968).

15. A. R. Holt J.Hunt and B. L. Moisewitsch, Phys. **B4**, L41-3(1971).

16. B. R. Junker, Phys. Rev. A**11**, 1552(1975).

17. S. Geltman, J. Phys. B**4**, 1288(1971).

18. S. Geltman and M.B. Hidalgo, J. Phys. B**4**, 1299(1971).

19. X. M. Tong and C.D. Lin, J. Phys. B:At.Mol.Opt. Phys.**38**, 2593(2005).

20. P.G. Burke and K.A. Berrington Atomic and Molecular processes: A R-matrix approach(Bristol: institute of Physics Publishing) (1993).

21. C.J. Gillan, J. Tennyson and P.G. Burke, Computational Methods for Electron-Molecule Collision(ed) W.M. Huo and F.A. Gianturco(New York: Plenum)(1995).

22. K. L. Baluja, P. G. Burke and L. A. Morgan, Comput. Phys. Commun. **27** 299(1982).

23. L.A. Morgan Comput. Phys. Commun. **31** 419(1984).

24. L.A. Morgan, C.J. Gillan, J. Tennyson and X. Chen, J. Phys. B: At.Mol. Opt. Phys.**30** 4087 (1997).

25. L.A. Morgan, J. Tennyson and C. J. Gillan, Comput. Phys. Commun. **114,** 120(1998).

26. B.M. Nestmann, K. Plingst and S.D. Peterimhoff , J. Phys. B: At.Mol. Opt. Phys.**27**, 2297 (1994).

27. J. Tennyson, J. Phys. B: At.Mol. Opt. Phys.**29**, 6185 (1996).

28. A. Faure, J.D. Gorfinkiel, L.A. Morgan and J. Tennyson, Comput. Phys. Commun. **144** , 224(2002).

29. Z.Chen and A.Z. Msezane, J. Phys.B**35**, 815(2002).

30. N. Anderson and K. Barschat, J. Phys.B**35**, 4507(2002).

31. G. X. Chen, A. K. Pradhan and W. Eissner, J. Phys. B**36**, 453(2003).

32. K. Barschat, O. Zatsarinny, I. Bray, D.V. Fursa and A. T. Stelbovics, J. Phys. B**37**, 2617(2004).

33. K.Muktawat, R. Srivastava and A. D. Stauffer, J. Phys. B**37**, 2165(2004).

34. B. Predojevic, D. Sevic, V. Pejcev, B. P. Marinkovic and D. M. Flipovic, J. Phys. B**38**, 1329(2005).

35. K. A. Berrington, C. P. Balance, D. C. Griffin and N. R. Badnell, J. Phys. B**38**, 1667(2005).

36. A. B. Voitkiv, Phy.Rev. A **72**, 062705(2005).

37. Rajesh Srivastava, A.D. Stauffer and Lalita Sharma, Phys. Rev. A**74**, 012715(2006).

38. J. Christopher Fontes and Hong Lin Zhang, Phy.Rev. A **76**, 040703(2007).

39. Yasuyuki Ishikawa, Phys. Rev. A **77**, 052701 (2008).

40. N. R. Badnell, J. Phys. B: At. Mol. Opt. Phys. **41**, 175202 (2008).

41. Jasmeet Singh Rajvanshi and K. L. Baluja, Phys. Rev. A **84**, 042711 (2011).

42.   M.A. Khakoo *et al*, Phys.Rev. A**65**, 062711(2002).

43.   W. M. Ariyasinghe and C. Goains, Phys. Rev. A **70**, 052709 (2004).

44.   M. Allan, Phys. Rev. A**74**, 030701 (2006).

45.   M. A. Stevenson and B. Lohmann, Phys. Rev. A**77**, 032708(2008).

46.   M. Hashino, H. Hoto, H. Tanaka, I. Bray, D.V. Fursa and S.J. Buckman, J. Phys. B: At.Mol. Opt. Phys.**42,** 145202 (2009).

47.   Peter Caradonna, James P. Sullivan and Adric Jones, Phys. Rev. A**80**, 060701(2009).

48.   Lukasz Klosowski, Mariusz Piwinski, Dariusz Dziczek, Katarzyna Pleskacz, and Stanislaw Chwirot, Phys.Rev. A **80**, 062709 (2009).

49.   M. A. Stevenson, L. R. Hargreaves, B. Lohmann, I. Bray, D. V. Fursa, K. Bartschat and A. Kheifets, Phys. Rev. A **79**, 012709 (2009).

50.   R.Ward, D. Cubric, N. Bowring, G. C. King, F. H. Read, D. V. Fursa, I. Bray, O. Zatsarinny and K. Bartschat, J. Phys. B: At. Mol. Opt. Phys. **44,** 045209(2011).

51.   A.C.L. Jones, C. Makochekanwa, P. Caradonna, D.S Slaughter, J.R. Machacek, R.P. McEachran, J.P. Sullivan and S.J. Buckman, Phys.Rev. A**83**, 032701(2011).

52.   A. Zecca *et al*, J. Phys. B: At.Mol. Opt. Phys.**45**, 015203 (2012).

53.   X. M. Tong and C.D. Lin, J. Phys. B: At. Mol. Opt. Phys. **38**, 2593(2005).

CHAPTER-2

GROUND STATE EXCITATION OF HELIUM

2.1 INTRODUCTION

Electron impact excitation of atoms is an essential aspect of atomic physics because it provides complete knowledge of atomic structure and processes. The measurements, in which inelastically scattered electron and radiated photons are detected in coincidence experiments, exploit the role of symmetry in scattering process by observing planer rather than axial symmetry. This feature enables observations of the non-spherical distortions, and rotational properties of electron charge cloud in the excited state as a function of scattering dynamics. When an electron collides with an atom or molecule, many processes can take place (excitation, ionization, dissociation, *etc.*), and the probability of a particular process taking place is characterized by its cross section. The knowledge of these cross sections is of great importance in many branches of physics; this is why excitation of atoms by electron impact has created increasing interest among the theoreticians and experimental workers providing a framework containing various information about projectile and target. The study of excitation processes by electron and positron impact is important for better understanding of matter and the anti-matter interactions and also for numerous applications. Electron scattering contributed significantly to the formulation of quantum wave mechanics and provide new insight into atomic structure. The excitation of rare gases is an important mechanism in a wide variety of phenomena. The accurate cross sections for electron impact excitation of rare gases are important for modeling and understanding processes that occur in gas discharge lasers, industrial plasmas, astrophysical plasmas, and electron-beam pumped lasers.

The collision of electrons with Helium atom is one of the most intensely studied atomic interactions giving a fertile testing ground for the investigation of fundamental processes. Experimentally, Helium is inert and easy to work with. From the theoretical standpoint, Helium is simplest atom for which there are no exact wavefunction or atomic potential. Consequently this collision target is testing ground for theoretical and experimental methods by becoming a standard case for evaluating the validity of collision theory as a three-electron system. This is particularly true for an appreciation of the exchange interaction and also for typical electron-correlation phenomena. From an applied perspective, knowledge of these cross sections is essential in the design of fusion reactors too. This follows as Helium is produced as a by-product (usually called 'ash') in the fusion reactor, which can then contribute as one of the important plasma-temperature loss processes in the reactor. Therefore it is worthwhile providing a reliable database of Helium cross sections so that all the effects can be accounted. With its relatively simple electronic structure Helium has been invaluable for developing our knowledge of few-body atomic interactions. As an inert atomic gas at room temperature, it is also particularly amenable to high-precision measurement, and electron-impact collisions with its two valence electrons provides a rich set of three and four-body interaction channels. Three-body interactions include elastic, single-excitation, and single-ionization collisions.

Electron scattering has historically been a preferred tool for interrogating the structure and other properties of the matter. In this view, here we are interested in the interaction of electron with Helium. Janssen and Norman Lockyer in 1868 detected Helium gas in the sun's atmosphere from their spectroscopic observation. The element was named Helium by Lockyer and Frankland after Helios, the Greek word for sun. Ramsey found the element in 1895 in a sample of cleveite, a Uranium mineral, after removing nitrogen and oxygen by treatment with sulfuric acid. The examination of the spectrum showed a yellow line for Helium along with the spectral line for Argon. Swedish chemists Cleve and Langlet also discovered Helium in mineral Uranium. Helium occurs in great abundance in all stars in the universe. Except for Hydrogen, it is the second most abundant element in the universe. Stars derive their energy from thermonuclear conversion of Hydrogen into Helium. Our sun is composed of 20% Helium. However, in the earth's atmosphere Helium is present only in trace amounts, 5.24 ppm. Its abundance in the earth's crust is only 8g/kg. In seawater, it occurs at a concentration of $0.007\mu g/L$. The origin of Helium on earth is attributed to alpha decay of Uranium, Thorium and other radioactive materials in the earth's crust. An alpha particle is a single charged Helium ion, He^+, which readily converts into a Helium atom in its passage through the earth's crust. Helium occurs in varying concentrations in many natural gas fields. In the United States, some natural gas deposits are found to contain Helium at up to 8% by volume, mostly associated with Nitrogen and hydrocarbon gases. Helium has several important industrial applications in analytical chemistry, metallurgy, space research, medicine, and low-temperature super cooling. Liquid Helium is used as a cryogenic fluid for super cooling and low temperature cooling baths. Helium-3 is used as a circulating medium in laboratory refrigerators to maintain constant temperatures below $3°K$. Gaseous Helium is used as a carrier for gas chromatographic analysis and as a purging gas for measuring volatile organics. It is used as a lifting gas in buoyant airships and in most types of balloons, such as weather, toy, kite-type, and advertising balloons. Its lifting power is just slightly less that of Hydrogen. In metallurgy, Helium is used to provide an inert atmosphere for growing crystals of high purity Silicon and Germanium for making transistors and diodes; as an inert shield for arc welding of metals; and to sparge dissolved gas from molten metals during purifications. In nuclear physics, Helium ions or alpha particles serve as projectiles in bombarding heavy nuclei to produce energy or to obtain artificial radioisotopes. It also is used for heat transfer and coolant in nuclear reactors. Some other applications of Helium include: detecting leaks in pressure containers and high-vacuum equipment; in lasers; in luminous signs for advertising; to fill space between lenses in optical instruments non-reactively; to provide an inert atmosphere for chemical reactions in the absence of air; to displace fuels and oxidizers from storage tanks in rockets or to introduce fuels into combustion chambers under Helium pressure; as a non-nitrogen diluent for Oxygen in SCUBA diving (so divers avoid the bends); and to mix with oxygen for treatment of respiratory diseases. Liquid Helium is used in magnetic resonance imaging (MRI) equipment for diagnosis of cancer and other soft tissue diseases. During last twenty years electron (positron)-Helium collision problem has been one of the most studied subject matter in the atomic and molecular collision physics due to its applications discussed above. It is still currently a very rapidly expanding field theoretically as well as experimentally. The reason is partly due to the development of highly sophisticated experimental technology with which one can study in a realistic manner the very complex nature of the collision dynamics involved and partly the easy access to fast speed computers with which one can perform cumbersome calculations in a short time. The studies on the electron impact excitation of the 2^1S and 3^1S state from the ground 1^1S state in Helium atom are interesting because these processes are typical example of transitions between the states for which the term symbols are the same for initial and final states. In last decade a number of experimental and theoretical results have been reported by on electron impact excitation of Helium. There is however, little agreement exist among the various results.

Bartschat and Andersen [1] have been reported electron impact excitation of Helium 3^1D state. They also reported the channel-coupling effects on the orientation. Plottke et al [2] have been used the Laguurre based convergent close coupling method to calculate electron impact excitation of the auto-ionizing states as well as other cross sections for scattering from the $1^1S,2^1S$ and 2^3S initial states of Helium. The calculations are done with S-wave model. Elazzouzi et al [3] have been reported angular distribution for Helium by electron impact at low incident energy. Using S-wave model electron-impact excitation and ionization of Helium is studied by Horner *et al* [4]. They used a time-dependent formulation of the exterior complex scaling method that does not involve the solution of large linear systems of equations and then presented total excitation, total ionization, and single differential cross sections from the ground and $n = 2$ excited states by comparing their results with those obtained by others using a frozen-core model. Colgan *et al* [5] used the time-dependent close-coupling method to calculate total integral, single differential, double differential, and triple differential ionization cross sections of Helium for impact electron energies ranging from 32 to 45 eV. For all quantities, the calculated cross sections are found to be in very good agreement with experiment, and for the triple differential cross sections, good agreement is also found with calculations made using the convergent close-coupling technique. Ralchenko *et al* [6] have evaluated cross section data for excitation of Helium and presented it by analytic fit function which preserves the correct asymptotic behavior of cross sections. Harris *et al* [7] have discussed the importance of projectile interactions in DCS for simultaneous excitation-ionization of Helium using distorted wave model. Excitation(differential and integeral) cross section, total cross sections and ionization cross sections for electron scattering on the metastable level 2^1S of Helium have been calculated by Wang etal [8] at low and intermediate energies. Further a propagating exterior complex scaling (PECS) method is developed and applied by Bartlett and Stelbovics [9] to the electron-impact of Helium in an *S*-wave model. Time-independent solutions to the Schrodinger equation are found numerically over a wide range of energies and used to evaluate total and differential cross sections for a complete set of three- and four-body processes with benchmark precision. In this model they have demonstrated the suitability of the PECS method for the complete solution of the full electron-Helium system exploring the details of theoretical and computational development of the four-body PECS method for three-body channels: single excitation and single ionization. Kartono and Mamat [10] have been calculated differential and total cross section for elastic and excitation from the ground state to n $\leq$ 2 states of atomic Helium by electrons for incident energies from 5 to 50 eV using close coupling-expansion. In the direct application, Zammit *et al* [11] have investigated electron-Helium scattering in weakly coupled hot-dense (Debye) plasma using the convergent close-coupling method. The Yukawa-type Debye-Huckel potential has been used to describe plasma Coulomb screening effects. Benchmark results are presented for momentum transfer cross sections, excitation, ionization, and total cross sections for scattering from the ground and metastable states of Helium. The calculations covered the entire energy range up to 1000 eV for the no screening case and various Debye lengths (5–100 a_0).They found the increase in screening interaction and total ionization cross sections while decrease in the excitation and total cross sections. Harris *et al* [12] have presented fully differential cross section (FDCS) calculations for electron-impact excitation and ionization of Helium using the four body distorted wave-exchange (4DWE) model. This model includes both the direct and exchange amplitudes, which account for the indistinguishability of the free electrons in the final state. The results of the 4DWE model are compared with absolute experimental results, and they found that the exchange amplitude has a minimal impact in determining the shape and magnitude of the FDCS. Zatsarinny and Bartschat [13] have presented cross sections for electron-impact ionization and simultaneous ionization plus excitation of Helium by electron impact by fully nonperturbative close-coupling formalism using B-spline R-matrix approach which contains a number of pseudostates in the expansion of the wave function. Recently differential and integral cross sections for the excited states 1s2p 3P, 1s3s 3S, 1s3p 3P and 1s3d 3D of Helium from the metastable state 1s2s 3S are calculated by Yanga *et al* [14] using the relativistic distorted wave method. A systematical comparison is made with the available experimental and theoretical results and better agreement is found when the results are compared with previous calculations and experiments for the integral cross sections. For differential cross sections, their results are in general agreement with the experimental data compared with the previous theoretical values.

With the help of moveable target method a group of California State University has developed [15] and measured Normalized doubly differential cross sections for the electron-impact ionization of Helium at energies 26.3, 28.3, 30.3, 32.5, 34.3, 36.5, and 40.7 eV and for scattering angles of $10°$–$130°$. Their results show very good quantitative agreement with the convergent close coupling calculations and are expected to be more improved in future. A new experimental technique has been applied by Lange *et al* [16] to measure absolute scattering cross sections for electron impact excitation of the $n = 2, 3$ states of Helium at near-threshold energies. The experimental results are compared with predictions from recent theoretical calculations. The calculations are performed using the *R*-matrix with pseudostates, *B*-spline *R*-matrix, and the convergent close-coupling methods. Generally, very good agreement is found between the experiment and the three theories. Using a high-sensitivity toroidal electron spectrometer, Bellm *et al* [17] have measured cross-section ratios for transitions leading to the first three excited states of the residual Helium ion relative to the transition leaving the ion in the ground state. Measurements are performed for both symmetric and asymmetric energy sharing kinematics. By presenting results as a ratio, a direct comparison is made between theoretical and experimental predictions without recourse to normalization. The experimental data are compared to theoretical predictions employing various first-order models and a second-order hybrid distorted wave plus convergent *R* matrix with pseudostates (close-coupling) approach. An electron momentum spectroscopy study on ionization-excitation processes of He is reported by Watanable *et al* [18]. The symmetric noncoplanar (*e,2e*) cross sections for transitions to excited states have been measured relative to that to the ground state at impact energies of 1240 and 4260 eV. Their experimental results exhibit a marked dependence on the impact energy providing strong evidence of involved higher-order effects. Further, Ward *et al* [19] have been measured the differential cross sections (DCS) for inelastic electron scattering to the $n = 2$ states in Helium at incident energies of 80, 100 and 120 eV. These DCS have been determined across the complete angular scattering range (0–180^0) using a magnetic angle changer (MAC) with a soft-iron core. An agreement between the experimental data and the predictions from these highly sophisticated theoretical methods is generally good. The remaining discrepancies mainly occur at small and large angles for the triplet states 2^3S and 2^3P, whereas excellent agreement is found between 30^0 and 150^0. The $(e,2e)$ cross sections for transitions to the $n=1$, 2, and 3 final state of He^+ have been measured by Ren *et al* [20] at impact energies of 1000 and 1600 eV by using a newly developed energy and momentum dispersive spectrometer. Binding energy spectra in the range of 8 to 86 eV and momentum profiles for the transitions to the ground and excited ion states of He^+ are reported at different impact energies and the experimental results are compared with plane wave impulse approximation calculations. The impact energy dependence of cross section ratios for the He^+ $n=1$, 2, and 3 final states are obtained. They observed some discrepancies between experimental data and theoretical calculations. Stevenson and Lohmann [21] have presented fully differential measurements of 730 eV electron-impact single ionization of the ground state of Helium with 205 and 100 eV outgoing electrons with the help of electron-electron coincidence spectrometer using coplanar asymmetric kinematics. Inter normalized data are obtained for coplanar geometries with the fast electron detected at $\theta_A = 6°, 9°,$ and 12°. They compared their data, where possible, with the corresponding data of Catoire *et al* [22] and the convergent close-coupling theory. An improved agreement is found between the present measurements and the theory. Hoshino *et al* [23] have presented normalized experimental differential cross sections and theoretical close coupling approximation data for electron impact excitation of the $n = 2$ states in Helium. The incident electrons have energies in the range 23.5–35 eV, while the scattered electrons are detected over the angular range 10^0–130^0. Agreement between their measured and calculated

DCS is generally good, often to better than 15%, with both also being in good accord with the available earlier measurements. Recently electron impact coherence parameters for inelastic electron Helium scattering have been measured by Klosowski *et al* [24]   for the excitation to the 2^1P state at collision energy of 100 eV. The experiment is conducted using angular correlation electron-photon coincidence technique with a magnetic angle changer allowing measurements in full range of scattering angles. The results are compared with other experimental data and theoretical predictions available for this collisional system.

2.2 THEORY

The scattering of electrons from atoms can be well represented as a potential scattering problem by including the static and polarization potentials as well as exchange in the case of electrons. Above the thresholds, the existence of additional exit channels for the incident particle flux means that simple potential scattering models produce an overestimate of the elastic cross sections. More elaborate theories, such as the convergent close coupling [25] or *R*-matrix [26] methods, take into account these additional channels but at the cost of a very substantial increase in the complexity of the problem and computer resources needed, this is why we are needed to treat the problems above threshold by such high energy methods one of which Pseudostate-Close-Coupling is considered here.

The time independent Schrödinger equation for electron scattering from atomic Helium is-

$$(E - H)|\Psi(x_0, x_1, x_2)\rangle = 0 \qquad\qquad \text{.... (2.1)}$$

where the Hamiltonian

$$H = H_T + H_0 + V_{01} + V_{02} \qquad\qquad \text{.... (2.2)}$$

Here subscripts 0, 1 & 2 are used to denote the projectile and target electrons respectively. H_T is the Hamiltonian target operator. The electron-electron potentials are V_{01} and V_{02}. To solve this equation, we write $|\Psi\rangle$ as explicitly anti-symmetrized wave functions utilizing the multichannel expansion.

$$|\Psi(x_0, x_1, x_2)\rangle = (1 - P_{01} - P_{02}) \sum \int_n |\phi_n(x_1, x_2) f_n(x_0)\rangle \qquad \text{.... (2.3)}$$

Where P_{01} and P_{02} are the space (coordinate and spin) exchange operators. To derive the close coupling equations, we obtain the complete set of target states by solving

$$H_T |\phi_n\rangle = \varepsilon_n |\phi_n\rangle \qquad \text{.... (2.4)}$$

where the completeness relation for the states is expressed as

$$I = \sum \int_n |\phi_n(x_1, x_2)\rangle\langle\phi_n(x_1, x_2)| \qquad \text{.... (2.5)}$$

with the subscripts indicating the electron space. The index n is discrete for negative energies and continuous for positive energies.

By inserting the eigenfunctions expansion we obtain close coupling (CC) equation as

$$\sum \int_n (K_0 \delta_{mn} + V_{mn}) f_n = (E - \varepsilon_m) f_m \qquad \text{.... (2.6)}$$

Where

$$V_{mn} = \langle\phi_m|V|\phi_n\rangle;$$

$$V = V_0 + V_{01} + V_{02} + (E - H)(P_{01} + P_{02}) \qquad \text{.... (2.7)}$$

The CC equations may be written more compactly as

$$(G_0^{-1}(E) - V(E)|f\rangle = 0 \qquad \text{.... (2.8)}$$

where G_0 is the operator with matrix elements

$$(G_0(E))_{mn} = \delta_{mn}(E - \varepsilon_m - K_0)^{-1} \qquad \text{.... (2.9)}$$

And $|f\rangle$ is the column vector whose components are the f_n .

Using the Green's function, differential form of the coupled equations can be solved for f_n and finally we obtain Lippmann-Schwinger (LS) equation. The LS equation for the system is

$$|f_n\rangle = |n\vec{k}_n\rangle + G_0(E^{(+)})V|f_n\rangle \qquad \text{.... (2.10)}$$

And $|n\vec{k}_n\rangle_m \equiv \delta_{mn}\,\phi_n|\vec{k}_n\rangle$ is the incident channel asymptotic state wave function. We adopt the Green's function $G_0(E^{(+)})$ which ensures outgoing spherical wave boundary conditions. In practice, it is more useful to use a LS equation for the T-matrix operator which we have formally defined by

$$|f_n\rangle = [1 + G_0(E^{(+)})T\,E^{(+)}]|n\vec{k}_n\rangle \qquad \text{.... (2.11)}$$

It is easy to check that the LS equation for T-matrix becomes

$$T(E^{(+)}) = V(E) + V(E)G_0(E^{(+)})T(E^{(+)}) \qquad \text{.... (2.12)}$$

The momentum-space matrix elements of the T-operator are

$$\langle m\vec{p}_m|T(E^{(+)})|n\vec{p}_n\rangle = \langle \vec{p}_m|T_{mn}(E^{(+)})|\vec{p}_n\rangle \qquad \text{.... (2.13)}$$

In order to solve the integral equation the momenta $\vec{p}_m$ & $\vec{p}_n$ are allowed to take on all possible values. The scattering amplitudes are derived from the on-shell amplitudes for which $\vec{p}_n = \vec{k}_n$ and $\varepsilon_n + \frac{1}{2}k_n^2 = \varepsilon_m + \frac{1}{2}k_m^2 = E$.

The criterion to apply the relation (13) is

$$\langle \phi_m|f_n\rangle = (-1)^S \langle \phi_n|f_m\rangle\,, \quad n, m = 1 \ldots\ldots N \qquad \text{.... (2.14)}$$

This identity is a result of applying the symmetry property of the wave functions to its CC expansion. The result of applying the new symmetry condition liberally is to modify the form of the exchange potential to the extent that there are no homogeneous solutions in the new forms LS equations [27]. In the anti-symmetrized two-electron basis of Hamiltonian, a radial part of the single particle functions ϕ_{nl} are taken as non orthogonal Laguerre-L^2 basis given by

$$\phi_{nl}(r) = (\lambda_l r)^{l+1} \exp(-\lambda_l r) \, L_n^{2l+1}(\lambda_l r) \qquad \text{.... (2.15)}$$

where the $L_n^{2l+1}(\lambda_l r)$ are associated Laguerre polynomials, λ_l is the interaction parameter and n ranges from 1 to the basis size N.

The target Hamiltonian H_T is

$$H_T = H_1 + H_2 + V_{12} \qquad \text{.... (2.16)}$$

Where

$$H_i = K_i + V_i = -\frac{1}{2}\nabla_i^2 - \frac{Z}{r_i} \qquad \text{.... (2.17)}$$

$for \; i = 1,2$, is the Hamiltonian of the He atom $(Z = 2)$, and

$$V_{12} = \frac{1}{r_{12}} \qquad \text{.... (2.18)}$$

is the electron-electron potential. Atomic units (a. u.) are assumed throughout.

For the target, Frozen core approximation is taken *i.e.* first electron of target is taken in lowest orbit while second electron is described by set of independent L^2 functions. The resulting target states $\phi(x_1, x_2)$, where x is used to denote both the spatial and spin coordinates, satisfy

$$\left\langle \phi_m \left| -\frac{1}{2}\nabla_1^2 - \frac{Z}{r_1} - \varepsilon_{n_\alpha} \right| \phi_n \right\rangle = 0 \qquad \text{.... (2.19)}$$

in order to get a good description of the He atom state, where ε_{n_α} is the energy associated with the $1s$ state of Helium atom. The excitation states for $\phi(x_1, x_2)$, can be obtained by solving the equation

$$\left\langle \phi_m \left| -\frac{1}{2}\nabla_2^2 - \frac{Z}{r_2} - \varepsilon_{n_\beta} \right| \phi_n \right\rangle = 0 \qquad \text{.... (2.20)}$$

where ε_{n_β} is the energy associated with the excitation states of the Helium atom.

After diagonalization of the ground and excitation states Hamiltonian, equations (2.19) and (2.20) can be written as the resulting three-term recurrence relations which are set of orthogonal polynomials having a non-empty continuous spectrum in addition to an infinite discrete spectrum. The three-term recurrence relations of the Pollaczek polynomials have complied with the positivity condition. These results, known as Favard's theorem, can be found in Kartono *et al* [28]. The behaviour of the nonorthogonal Laguerre-L^2 basis function in equation (2.15) is oscillatory and depends upon the number of basis size N and interaction parameter λ_l. In order to get a good description of the ground and excitation states, we determine the interaction parameter λ_l from the positivity condition. In our work we simplify the problem by using the frozen-core model, in which all configurations have one of the electrons occupying the lowest orbital. In order to get a good description of the ground states we take $\lambda_0 = 4$ for $n = 1$. This choice generates the He $1s$ orbital, which allows us to take into account short range correlations in the ground state, as well as being suitable for obtaining an accurate representation of excited discrete and continuum states. To obtain good nS excited states we take $\lambda_0 = 0.93$ for $n > 1$.

The configuration interaction coefficients $C_{Ni}^{(\alpha\beta)}$ are given by

$$\left(C_{Ni}^{(\alpha\beta)} \right)^2 = \frac{2^{2l}}{\pi} \frac{\lambda_l}{\left(1 - X_{Ni}^{(\alpha\beta)}\right)} W_{Ni}^{(\alpha\beta)} \qquad \dots (2.21)$$

where the notations α and β are used to denote the first and second electron and W_{Ni} are the associated quadrature weights of Gaussian quadrature based Pollaczek polynomials which are given by

$$W_{Ni}^{(\alpha\beta)} = \frac{\pi \Gamma(N + 2l + 1)}{2^{2l}\Gamma(N+1)} \frac{1}{P_{N-1}^{l+1}\left(X_{Ni}^{(\alpha\beta)}\right) \dfrac{d\, P_N^l\left(X_{Ni}^{(\alpha\beta)}\right)}{dx}}$$

$$\dots (2.22)$$

This rearrangement is such that the asymptotic (large r_0) Hamiltonian is $K_0 + H_T$, and this will be used to generate the Green's functions and boundary conditions for the total wave functions

$$\lim_{r_0 \to \infty} \psi(x_0, x_1, x_2) = \chi(\sigma) \exp\left(i\vec{k}_i \cdot \vec{r}_0\right) \phi_i(x_1, x_2) \qquad \dots (2.23)$$

Where $\vec{k}_i$ is the incident projectile momentum and the incident projectile momentum and ϕ_i is the initial target state. The coupled LS equation for the T-matrix is

$$\langle \vec{k}_f^{(-)} \phi_f | T | \phi_i \vec{k}_f^{(+)} \rangle$$

$$= \langle \vec{k}_f^{(-)} \phi_f | V | \phi_i \vec{k}_i^{(+)} \rangle$$

$$+ \sum_n \int_n \int_k d^3k \, \frac{\langle \vec{k}_f^{(-)} \phi_f | V | \phi_n \vec{k} \rangle \langle \vec{k} \phi_n | T | \phi_i \vec{k}_i^{(+)} \rangle}{E^{(+)} - \varepsilon_n - k^2}$$

$$\dots (2.24)$$

where the projectile waves (discrete or continuous) k ($\pm$) satisfy the condition

$$\left(\varepsilon_k^{(\pm)} - K_0\right) | \vec{k}^{(\pm)} \rangle = 0 \qquad \dots (2.25)$$

The on-shell momenta $\varepsilon_k = {k_n^2}/{2}$ are obtained from

$$E - \varepsilon_n - k_n^2 = 0 \qquad \dots (2.26)$$

and exist only for open channels n such that $E = \varepsilon_i - {k_i^2}/{2} > \varepsilon_n$.

In solving the equation (2.24), the approach that is taken in this work is to diagonalize the Helium target Hamiltonian in a set of non-orthogonal Laguerre-L^2 basis function which when extended to completeness form a basis for the target Hilbert space. The use of non-orthogonal Laguerre-L^2 basis function eliminates the problem of singular continuum T-matrix elements raised during solution whenever i, f and n are in the continuum. Also most importantly, with a known basis the convergence of the expansions can be studied in a systematic manner with increasing number of basis functions.

We introduce a finite set of N square-integrable states $|\phi_n^N\rangle$ which satisfy

$$\langle\phi_m^N|H_T|\phi_n^N\rangle = \varepsilon_n^N \delta_{mn} \qquad\qquad\qquad\qquad ..... (2.27)$$

and have the property

$$\sum\int_n \phi_n(x_1,x_2)f_n(x_0) = \lim_{n\to\infty}\sum_{n=1}^{\infty}\phi_n^N(x_1,x_2)f_n^N(x_0) \qquad .... (2.28)$$

With these definitions, the sum and integral in (2.5) and the LS equation (2.24) become a single sum over N, with the target states and energies being replaced by $|\phi_n^N\rangle \varepsilon_n^N$, respectively. So instead of I, we define

$$I = \sum_{n=1}^{\infty}|\phi_n^N(x_1,x_2)\rangle\langle\phi_n^N(x_1,x_2)| \qquad\qquad .... (2.29)$$

And we have

$$\langle\vec{k}_f^{(-)}\phi_f^N|T|\phi_i^N\vec{k}_f^{(+)}\rangle$$

$$= \langle\vec{k}_f^{(-)}\phi_f^N|V|\phi_i^N\vec{k}_f^{(+)}\rangle$$

$$+ \sum_{n=1}^{N}\int_k d^3k \frac{\langle\vec{k}_f^{(-)}\phi_f^N|V|\phi_i^N\vec{k}_f^{(+)}\rangle\langle\vec{k}\phi_n^N|T|\phi_i^N\vec{k}_i^{(+)}\rangle}{E^{(+)} - \varepsilon_n^N - k^2}$$

$$.... (2.30)$$

where for the physical T-matrix elements of interest we must have $|\phi_f\rangle = |\phi_f^N\rangle$ and $|\phi_i\rangle = |\phi_i^N\rangle$ to sufficiently high precision. With these definitions we have

$$\langle k\phi_f|T|\vec{k}_i^{(+)}\phi_i\rangle = \lim_{n\to\infty}\langle k\phi_f^N|T|\vec{k}_i^{(+)}\phi_i^N\rangle \qquad\qquad .... (2.31)$$

for the physical T-matrix elements. The projection operator I is replaced by I^N in calculating the matrix elements of T-matrix. It is a Gaussian-type quadrature and the underlying orthogonal polynomials are of the Pollaczek class. It can be shown that weights of the negative energy L^2 states convergence to unity in equation (28) in the limit of large N. This ensures that the limiting procedure (2.31) gives the correct T-matrix amplitudes (2.24) for the transitions to $1S$, $2S$ and $2P$ levels.

The partial wave LS equation corresponding to (2.30) for the reduced T-matrix elements are

$$\langle L_f k_f^{(-)}, f\pi f^l f^S f \| T_{\pi S}^{JN} \| L_i k_i^{(+)}, i\pi_i l_i s_i \rangle$$

$$= \langle L_f k_f^{(-)}, f\pi f^l f^S f \| V_{\pi S}^{JN} \| L_i k_i^{(-)}, i\pi_i l_i s_i \rangle$$

$$+ \sum_{n=1}^{N} \sum_{l} \sum_{L} \sum_{k} \int \frac{\langle L_f k_f^{(-)}, f\pi f^l f^S f \| V_{\pi S}^{JN} \| L k^{(-)}, n\pi l s \rangle \langle L k^{(-)}, n\pi l s \| T_{\pi S}^{JN} \| L_i k_i^{(+)}, i\pi_i l_i s_i \rangle}{E^{(+)} - \varepsilon_n^N - \varepsilon_k}$$

$$\ldots\ (2.32)$$

The method of solving this equation is identical to the CCC method for hydrogen target [29].

The differential scattering cross section for scattering from channel i to channel f at an angle θ are given by

$$\frac{d\sigma_{fi}}{d\Omega} = (2\pi)^4 \frac{k_f}{k_i} \frac{\hat{S}^2}{\hat{l}^2} \sum_{m,L_i} \sum_{L_f, j} \left| \langle L_f K_f^{(-)} n_f, \pi_f, l_f, S_f \| T_{\pi S}^{JN} \| \langle L_i K_i^{(+)} n_i, \pi_i, i, S_i \right|^2$$

$$\ldots\ (2.33)$$

Total cross section (TCS) for excitation of He from an initial state i to final state f, is given by

$$\sigma_{i \to f} = \frac{2\pi}{k_i k_f} \int_{k_i - k_f}^{k_i + k_f} \left(\frac{d\sigma}{d\Omega} \right) \vec{q}\ dq \qquad \ldots\ (2.34)$$

Where $\vec{q}\ (= \vec{k_i} - \vec{k_f})$ is the momentum transfer vector.

2.3 RESULT AND DISCUSSION

We have calculated differential scattering cross section (DCS) for ground state excitation of atomic Helium at 100, 200 and 500 eV by electron impact using equation (2.33). Also, we have computed total scattering cross sections (TCS) of Helium using equation (2.34). Here the Pseudostate Close Coupling method is used with a non-orthogonal-L^2 basis for the 2^1S and 3^1S excited states. Our results along with other theoretical/experimental results for electron impact excitation of Helium atom from ground state to 2^1S and 3^1S states are presented in figures (2.1) to (2.8).

2.3.1 1^1S - 2^1S EXCITATION OF HELIUM

Figure (2.1) shows our result for the 1^1S - 2^1S excitation of Helium atom by electron impact at 100 eV. For comparison, we have plotted experimental results (E) of Chamberlain *et al* [30] and the outcome of second order diagonalization method (SODM) (S) used by Baye and Heenen [31]. From figure it can be seen that present result is in reasonable agreement with experimental data (E) up to entire angular range. The other theoretical result (S) gives higher DCS after 14^0 scattering angle.

Figure (2.2) shows our result for the same excitation of Helium atom by electron but at 200 eV. We have also plotted experimental results (E) of Chamberlain *et al* [30] and theoretical results of second order potential theory (SOPT) (S) used by Berrington *et al* [32]. Figure shows that present result is superior over S and best likeness with experimental result (E). The theoretical result (S) crosses the DCS at 10^0, while present results are in good agreement with experimental result up to 20^0 .

Figure (2.3) shows our result for the 1^1S - 2^1S excitation of Helium atom by electron at 500 eV. Here we have plotted the theoretical results of dipole corrected multichannel eikonal theory (DMET) (D) of Manksy and Flannery [33] and experimental results (E) of Skerbele and Lassettre [34]. From figure we observe that our result shows a very good agreement with the experimental data (E). The large angle region ($\theta > 13^0$), all results merge into each other. The DMET result show lower DCS upto 10^0.

Figure (2.4) shows our result of total scattering cross section (TCS) for the 1^1S - 2^1S excitation of Helium atom. For comparison, we have plotted the theoretical results using Born-exchange (BE) approximation [35]. We notice that our TCS is slightly greater than result obtained from Born exchange for whole angular range but both the TCS values tumble down simultaneously.

2.3.2   1¹S – 3¹S EXCITATION OF HELIUM

Figure (2.5) shows our result for the 1^1S - 3^1S excitation of Helium atom by electron at 100 eV. For comparison purpose, we have plotted the theoretical results (D) of Manksy and Flannery [33] obtained by DMET and generalized distorted wave method (GDWM) (G) of Winters *et al* [36]. It is evident from figure that DCS calculated by us lies in between G and D upto12^0 then after there is rapid decrease followed by rapid boost causing two bumps in result D relative to G. The results also emphasize the necessity of more sophisticated outcome due to not availability of experimental results.

Figure (2.6) shows our result for the 1^1S - 3^1S excitation of Helium atom by electron at 200 eV. For comparison, we have plotted the theoretical result (D) obtained by DMET of Manksy and Flannery [33] and GDWM (G) of Winters *et al* [36]. All the results closely agree only for a little range below 5^0, then D and G results are different but still they are comparable. At higher angle range ($\theta > 5^0$) our results are equally closed till the last value making it as average of results D & G.

Figure (2.7) shows our result for the 1^1S - 3^1S excitation of Helium atom by electron at 500 eV. For comparison, we have plotted the theoretical result of DMET used by Manksy and Flannery [33] and GDWM (G) of Winters *et al* [36]. From figure it is clear that after 5^0 there is little discrepancy among the results. No other experimental result is available for this transition at present to compare with our result and dominance to be proved over other.

Figure (2.8) shows our result of TCS for the 1^1S - 3^1S excitation of Helium atom. For comparison, we have plotted the theoretical results by Born-exchange approximation [35]. For this excited state same characteristics of result are found but at lower values of DCS as in the case of 2^1S excited state.

2.4 CONCLUDING REMARKS

In conclusion, our present calculations of angular dependence of DCS and energy dependence of TCS for excitations 1^1S-2^1S and 1^1S-3^1S are reproducing experimental and theoretical results well in same aspect. This is encouraging feature of the present calculations. Although, as we go towards the higher excited state and electron impact energy, an increasing discrepancy within a small shroud is seen specially after 5^0 scattering angle even the data are analogous. We expect that in near future calculations or measurements will have much higher precision both with regard to lower statistical error on the data and more through assessment of possible systematic errors.

FIGURE CAPTIONS

Figure [2.1] : **DCS for 1¹S - 2¹S Excitation of Helium by impact of electron at 100 eV**

———————— : Present result

.—.—.—.— : Experimental result (E) of Chamberlain *et al* [30]

- - - - - - - - - : Theoretical result (S) of Baye and Heenen [31]

Figure [2.2] : **DCS for 1¹S - 2¹S Excitation of Helium by impact of electron at 200 eV**

———————— : Present result

.—.—.—.— : Experimental result (E) of Chamberlain *et al* [30]

- - - - - - - - - : Theoretical result (S) of Berrington *et al* [32]

Figure [2.3] : **DCS for 1¹S - 2¹S Excitation of Helium by impact of electron at 500 eV**

———————— : Present result

.—.—.—.— : Experimental result (E) of Skerbele Lassettre [34]

- - - - - - - - - : Theoretical result (D) of Manksy and Flannery [33]

Figure [2.4] : **TCS for 1¹S - 2¹S Excitation of Helium by electron impact .**

———————— : Present result

.—.—.—.— : Born exchange (BE) approximation [35]

Figure [2.5]   : DCS for $1^1S - 3^1S$ Excitation of Helium by impact of electron at 100 eV

————————   : Present result

.—.—.—.—   : Theoretical result (G) of Winters *et al* [36]

- - - - - - - - - -   :Theoretical result (D) of Manksy and Flannery [33]

Figure [2.6]   : DCS for $1^1S - 3^1S$ Excitation of Helium by impact of electron at 200 eV

————————   : Present result

.—.—.—.—   : Theoretical result (G) of Winters *et al* [35]

- - - - - - - - - -   : Theoretical result (D) of Manksy and Flannery [33]

Figure [2.7]   : DCS for $1^1S - 3^1S$ Excitation of Helium by impact of electron at 500 eV

————————   : Present result

.—.—.—.—   : Theoretical result (G) of Winters *et al* [35]

- - - - - - - - - -   : Theoretical result (D) of Manksy and Flannery [33]

Figure [2.8]   : TCS for $1^1S - 3^1S$ Excitation of Helium by Electron impact

————————   : Present result

.—.—.—.—   : Born exchange (BE) approximation [35]

DCS FOR (1^{1}S - 2^{1}S) EXCITATION OF HELIUM BY IMPACT OF ELECTRON AT 100 eV

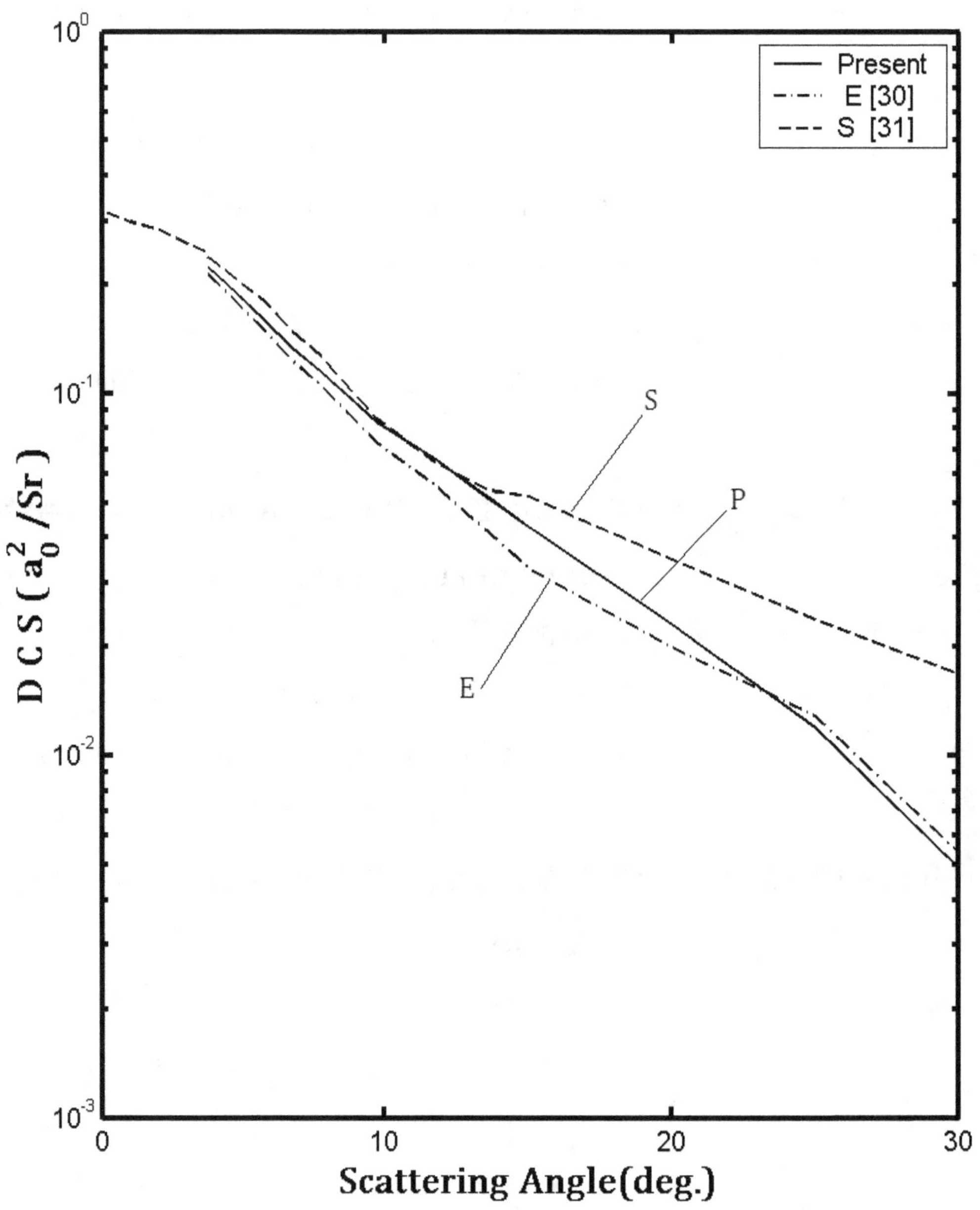

FIGURE [2.1]

DCS FOR (1¹S - 2¹S) EXCITATION OF HELIUM BY IMPACT OF ELECTRON AT 200 eV

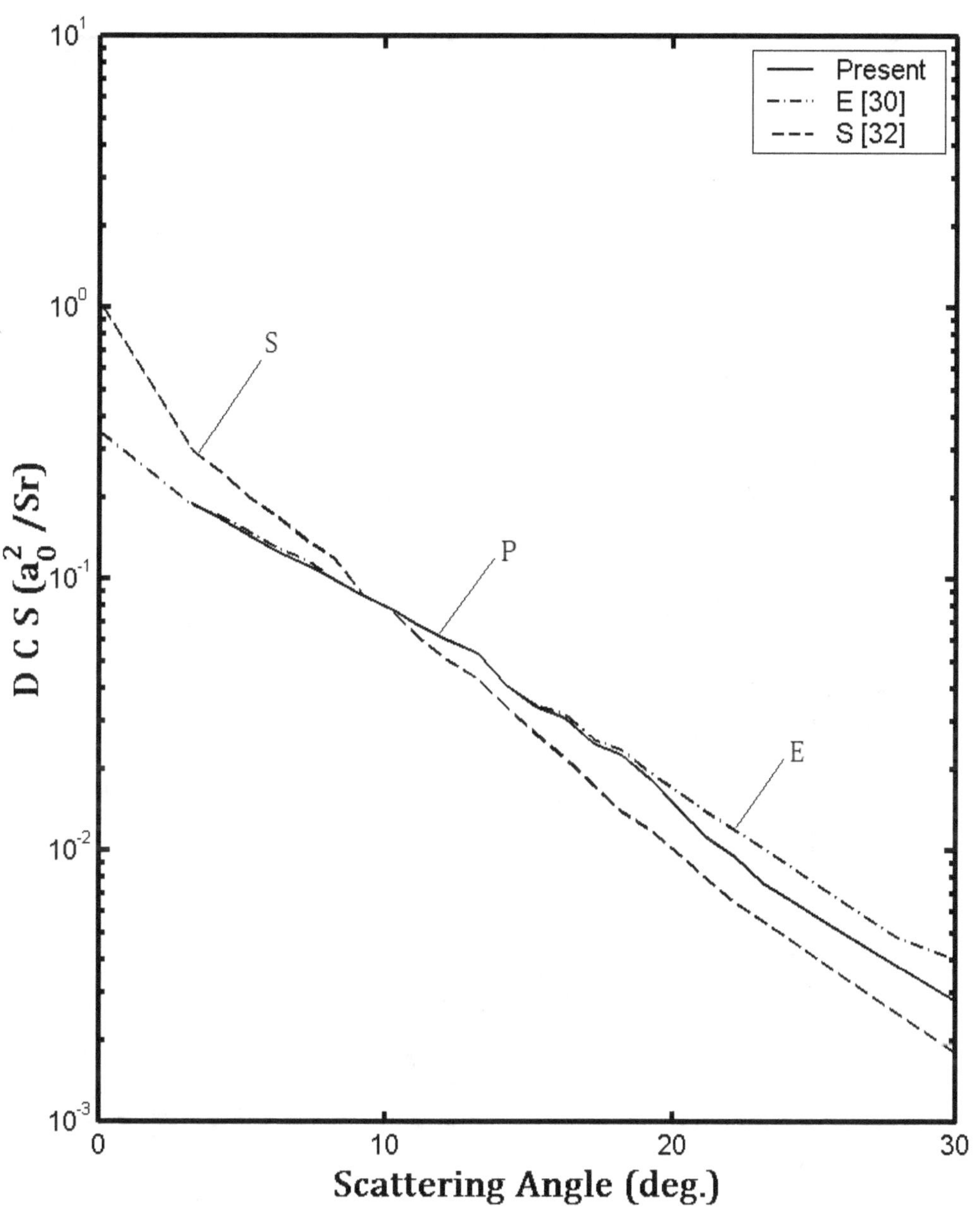

FIGURE [2.2]

DCS FOR (1¹S - 2¹S) EXCITATION OF HELIUM BY IMPACT OF ELECTRON AT 500 eV

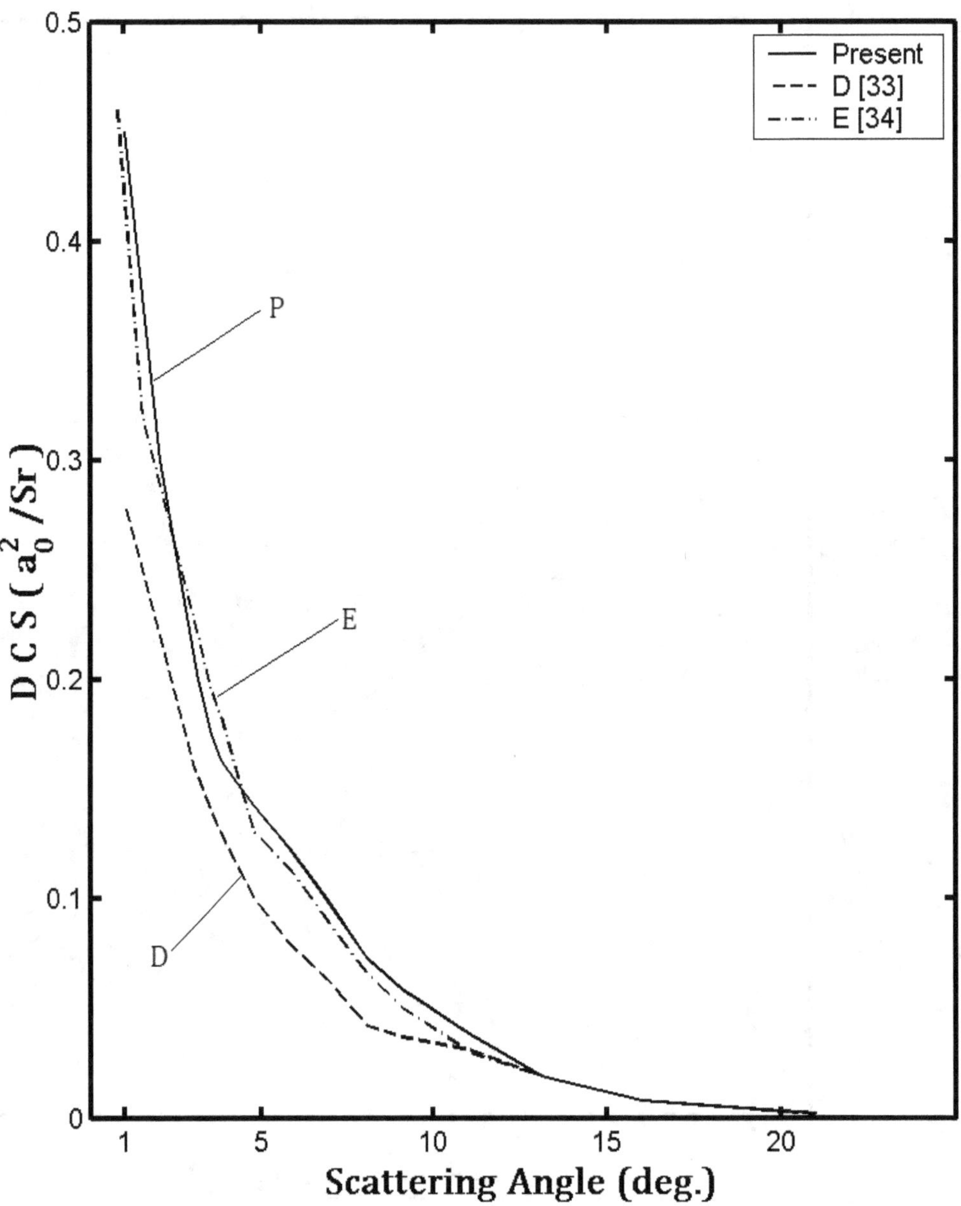

FIGURE [2.3]

TCS FOR (1¹S - 2¹S) EXCITATION OF HELIUM BY IMPACT OF ELECTRON

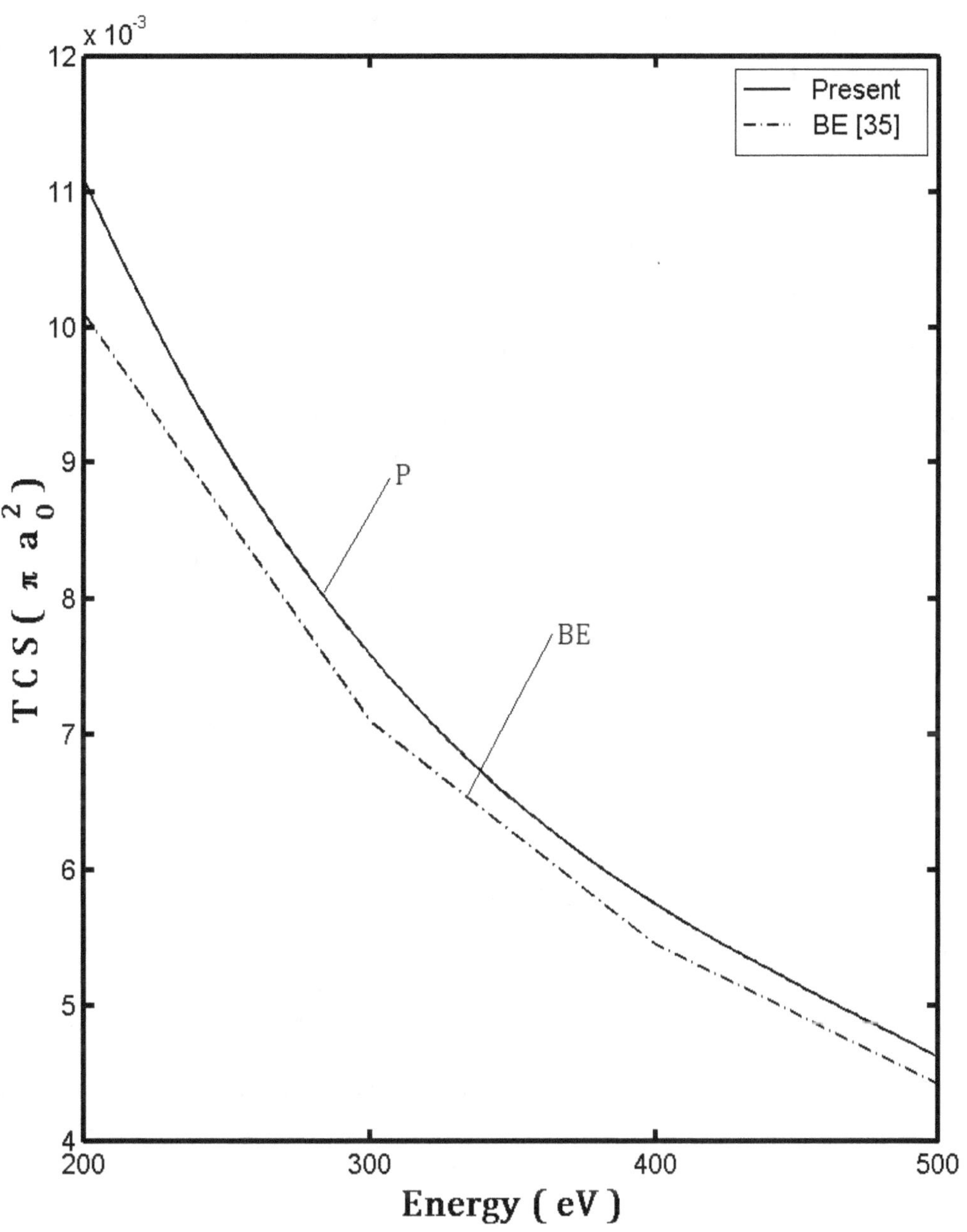

FIGURE [2.4]

DCS FOR (1¹S - 3¹S) EXCITATION OF HELIUM BY IMPACT OF ELECTRON AT 100 eV

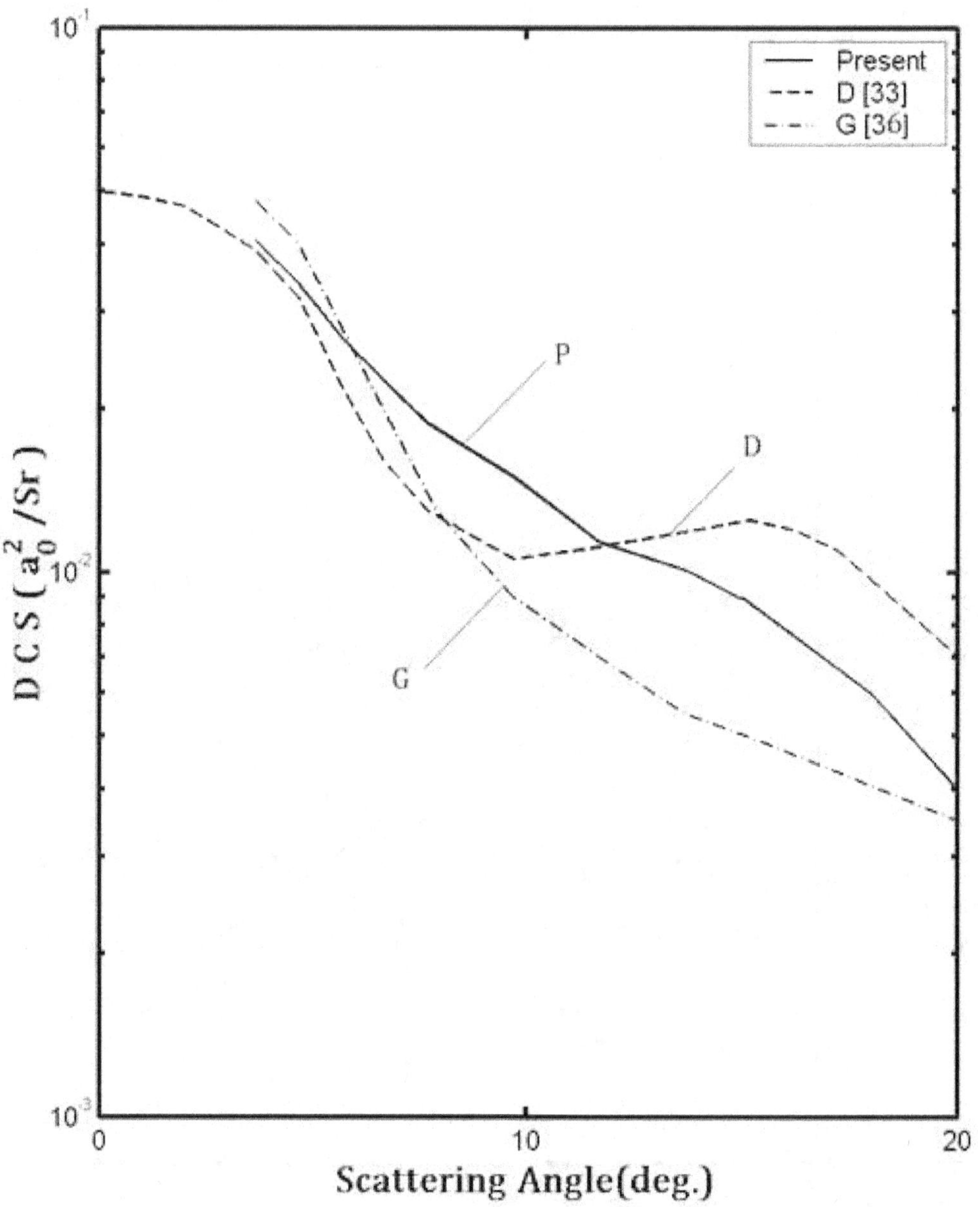

FIGURE [2.5]

DCS FOR (1¹S - 3¹S) EXCITATION OF HELIUM BY IMPACT OF ELECTRON AT 200 eV

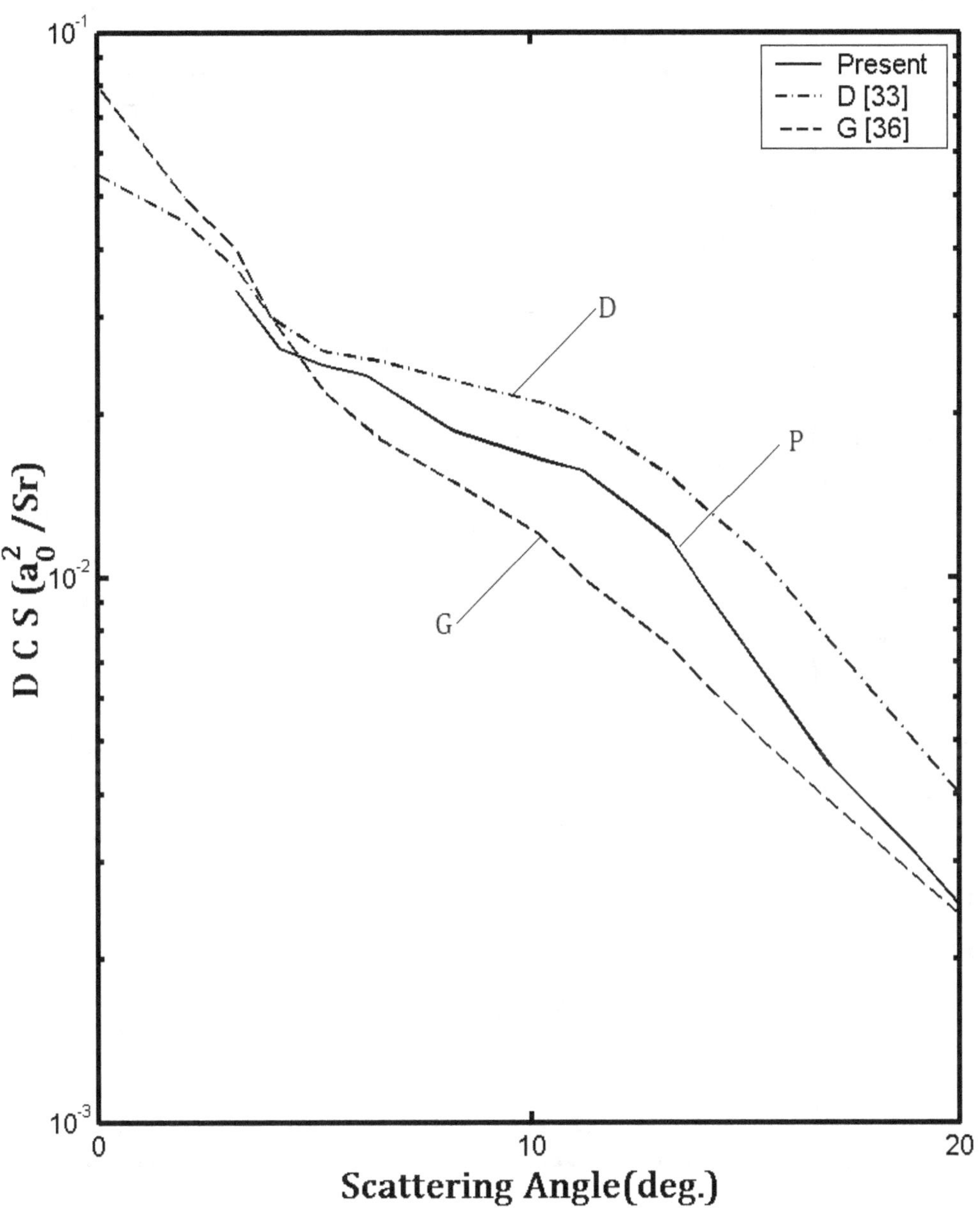

FIGURE [2.6]

DCS FOR (1¹S - 3¹S) EXCITATION OF HELIUM BY IMPACT OF ELECTRON AT 500 eV

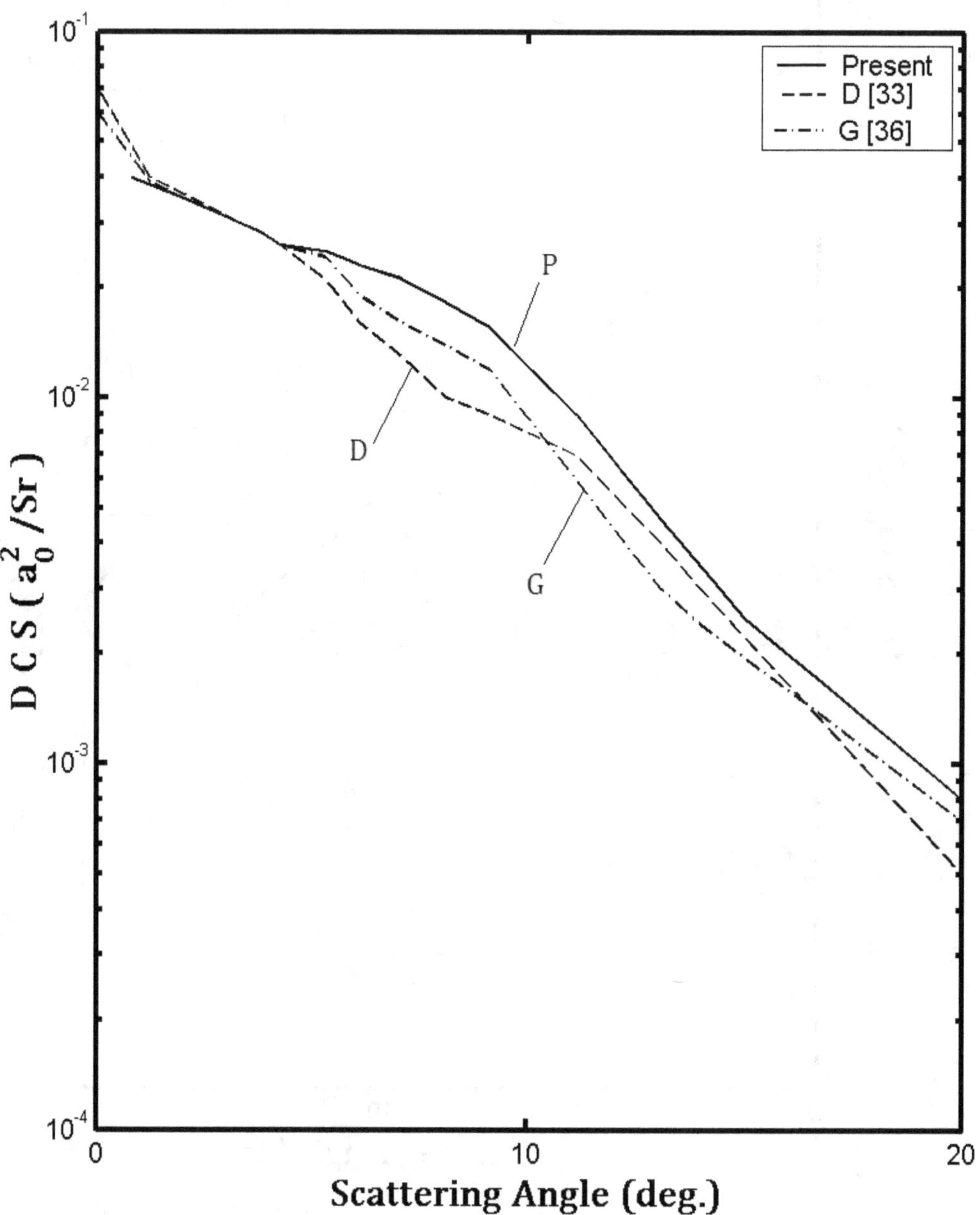

FIGURE [2.7]

TCS FOR (1¹S - 3¹S) EXCITATION OF HELIUM BY IMPACT OF ELECTRON

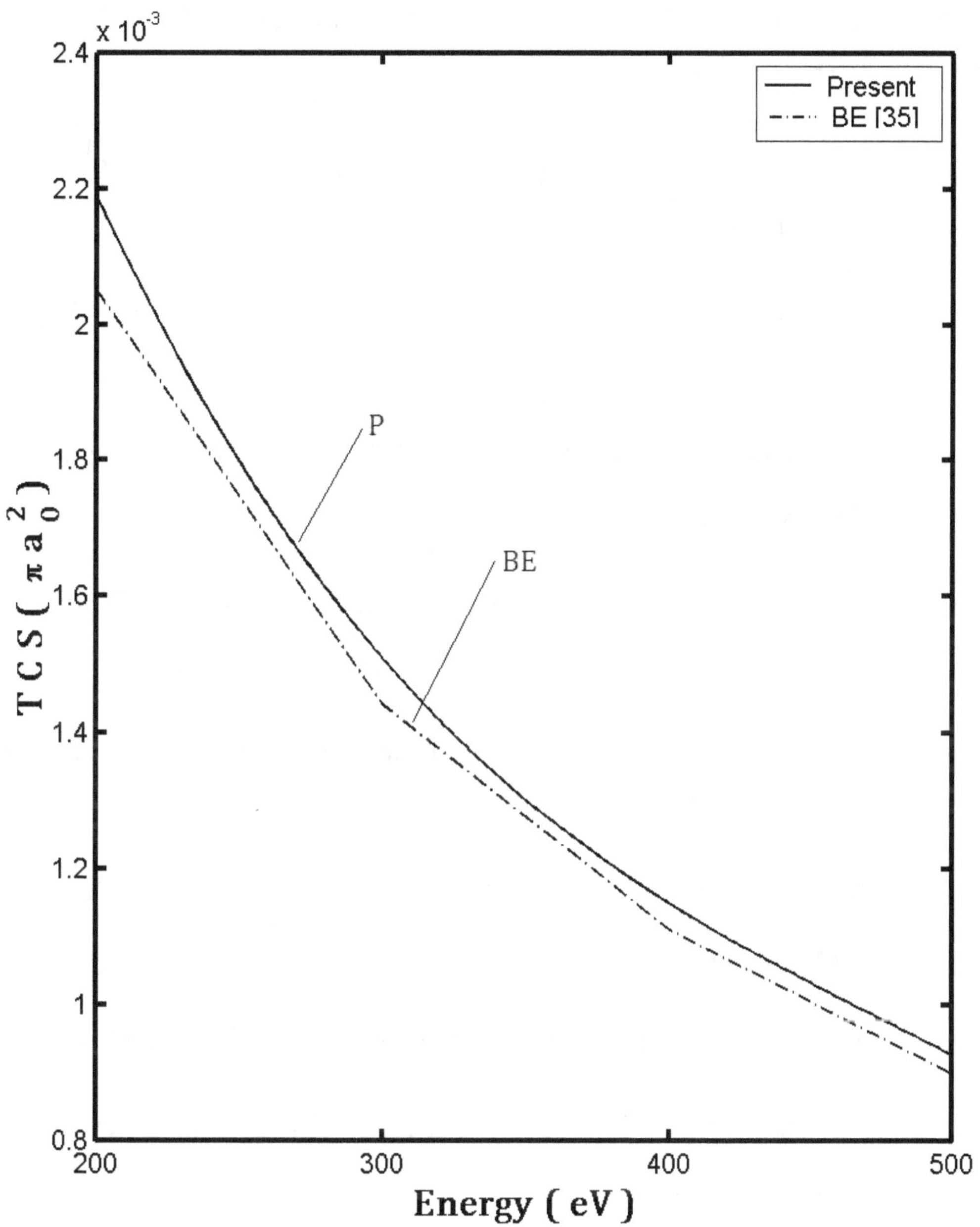

FIGURE [2.8]

<u>REFERENCES</u>

1. K. Bartschat and N. Andersen, J. of Phys. B**36**, 163(2003).

2. C. Plottke, P. Nicol, I. Bray, D. V. Fursa and A.T. Stelbovics, J. of Phys. B**37**, 3711(2004).

3. S. Elazzouzi, C. D. Cappello, A. Lahmam-Bennani and F. Catoire, J. of Phys. B**38**, 1391(2005).

4. D. A. Horner, C. William Mc Curdy, and T. N. Rescigno, Phys. Rev. A **71**, 012701 (2005).

5. J. Colgan, M. S. Pindzola, G. Childers, and M. A. Khakoo, Phys. Rev. A 73, 042710 (2006).

6. Yu. Ralchenko, R. K. Janev, T. Kato, D. V. Fursa, I. Bray, F. J. de Heer, Atomic Data and Nuclear Data Tables **94**, 603–622(2008).

7. L. Harris, M. Foster, Ciarm.-Ryan Anderson, J. L. Peacher and D.H. Madition, J. Phys. B**41**,135203(2008).

8. Y. C. Wang, Y. Zhou, Y, Cheng, K Ratnavelu and J. Ma, J. Phys. B**43**, 045201(2010).

9. P. L. Bartlett and Andris T. Stelbovics, Phys. Rev. A **81**, 022715 (2010).

10. A. Kartono and M. Mamat, Applied Mathematical Sciences, Vol. **4-27**, 1309 – 1328(2010).

11. M. C. Zammit, D. V. Fursa, I. Bray and R. K. Janev, Phys. Rev. A **84**, 052705 (2011).

12.   A. L. Harris, B. Milum, and D. H. Madison, Phy. Rev. A **84**, 052718 (2011).

13.   O. Zatsarinny and K. Bartschat, Phys. Rev. Lett. **107**, 023203(2011).

14.   N. X. Yanga, C. Z. Dongb, and J. Jiang, J. At. Mol. Sci. **3** 49-58(2012).

15.   E. Schow, K. Hazlett, J. G. Childers, C. Medina, G. Vitug, I. Bray, D. V. Fursa, and M. A. Khakoo, Phy. Rev. A **72**, 062717 (2005).

16.   M. Lange, J. Matsumoto, J. Lower, S. Buckman, O. Zatsarinny, K. Bartschat, I. Bray and D. Fursa, J. Phys. B: At. Mol. Opt. Phys. **39** 4179–4190(2006).

17.   S. Bellm, J. Lower, K. Bartschat, X. Guan, D. Weflen, M. Foster, A. L. Harris,and D. H. Madison, Phy. Rev. A **75**, 042704(2007).

18.   N. Watanabe, M. Takahashi, Y. Udagawa, K. A. Kouzakov and Yu. V. Popov, Phy. Rev. A **75**, 052701 (2007).

19.   R.Ward, D. Cubric, N. Bowring, G. C. King, F. H. Read, D. V. Fursa, I. Bray, O. Zatsarinny and K. Bartschat, J. Phys. B: At. Mol. Opt. Phys. **44 ,** 045209 (2011).

20.   X. G. Ren, C. G. Ning, J. K. Deng, G. L. Su, S. F. Zhang, Y. R. Huang, and G. Q. Li, Phys. Rev. A **72**, 042718 (2005).

21.   M. A. Stevenson and B. Lohmann, Phys. Rev. Λ **75**, 034701 (2007).

22.   F Catoire, E. M. Staicu-Casagrande, M. Nekkab, C. Dal Cappello, K. Bartschat and A. Lahmam-Bennani , J. Phys. B: At. Mol. Opt. Phys. **39**, 2827(2006).

23.   M. Hoshino, H. Kato, H. Tanaka, I. Bray, D. V. Fursa, S. J. Buckman,.O. Ingolfsson and M. J. Brunger J. Phys. B: At. Mol. Opt. Phys. **42 ,** 145202 (2009).

24.   L. Klosowski, M. Piwinski, D. Dziczek, K. Pleskacz, and S. Chwirot, Phy. Rev. A **80**, 062709(2009).

25.   I. Bray and Stelbovics , Phys. Rev. A **46,** 6995(1992).

26.   P. G. Burke , A. Hibbert and W. D. Robb, J. Phys. B: At. Mol. Phys. **4** 153(1971).

27.   A. T. Stelbovics and L. Berge, Phys. Rev. A. **55**, 1028-1038(1997).

28.   A. Kartono, T. Winata and Sukirno, Appl. Math. Comp., Elsevier, 879–893(2005).

29.   T. Winata and A. Kartono, Eur. Phys. J. D : At. Mol. Opt. Phys. **28,** 307-315. (2004).

30.   G. E. Chamberlain, S.R. Mielczarec and C.E. Kuyatt, , Phys. Rev. A **2,** 1905(1970).

31.   D. Baye and P. H. Heenen, , Phys. Rev. B **7,** 938(1974).

32.   K. A. Berrington, B. H. Bransden and J. P. Coleman, Phys. Rev. B **6,** 436(1973).

33.   E. J. Manksy and M. R. Flannery, Phys. Rev. B **23,** 4573(1990).

34.   A. Skerbele and E. N. Lassettre, J. chem.. Phys. **45**, 4077(1966).

35.   S. Saxena, Ph. D. thesis, (1984).

36.   K. H. Winters, M. Issa and B. H. Bransden, Can. J. phys.**55,** 1074(1977).

CHAPTER – 3

ELECTRON COLLISONAL EXCITATION OF NEON

3.1 INTRODUCTION

Electron scattering from the noble gases is an important problem in the field of atomic collisions. Numerous experimental and theoretical studies have been performed over many decades, both for fundamental and practical reasons. The detailed study of the many near-threshold resonance features [1] has proven to be very challenging to both experiment and theory alike and is valuable in the sense that it represents a sensitive test of the quality of new theoretical models. A reliable knowledge of elastic/inelastic cross sections for rare gases is very important in different valuable applications. The field of electron (positron) collision physics is needed to uncover and understand the broad range of dynamical processes that can occur when an electron or positron interacts with a complex atom. Many of the processes that have been uncovered to the date are now known to have a profound effect on the way in which some of everyday technological devices operate, and natural phenomena proceed. The elucidation of the dynamical aspects of scattering process is valuable because it is also important to understand the magnitude or rate with which they occur, in order to be able to quantify any possible applications. Measurements of scattering cross-sections and reaction rates are of critical importance across a range of scattering problems. In order to establish standards for such measurements, it is equally important that there be a series of benchmark measurements and calculations in the field, both as a standard for experimental and theoretical practice and as a guide for how theory may be applied to the many cases where experiments are intractable, for one reason or another. The investigation of electron/positron scattering from noble gases provides a vital meeting point for contemporary quantum scattering theory and experiment. The large amount of theoretical efforts applied to calculate various parameters attached to their importance. The accurate theoretical data provides the verification of experimental data as well as both side explanations of the mysteries. The noble gas systems are some of the simplest targets to study experimentally due to their inert nature and consequent ease of handling. With their closed valence shells they are also relatively simple collision systems to approach theoretically, although the level of complication increases with atomic number. Electron-atom scattering has been one of the most studied subjects in the atomic and molecular collision physics having many important applications. It is still currently a very rapidly expanding field theoretically and experimentally. The reason is partly due to the development of highly sophisticated experimental technology with which one can study in a realistic manner the very complex nature of the collision dynamics involved and partly the easy access to fast speed computers with which one can perform cumbersome calculations in a short time. The ability to calculate accurate elastic scattering cross sections in the noble gases represents a fundamental test of our understanding of the dynamics of electron atom interactions. It provides the basis upon which we can precede to open-shell atoms and to molecular systems.

In this work we aim to provide comparison between theoretical and experimental cross sections for atomic Neon gas targets that is more complex than Helium. We shall evaluate the theoretical view to establish an accepted set of cross sections for Neon gas target. Because of its stable heliumlike core, Neon appears over a wide range of astrophysical and laboratory plasma conditions. X-ray lines from Neon can be used as important temperature, density, and abundance diagnostics for these plasmas. In collisonal plasma, electron impact excitation is one of the main mechanisms for populating the upper levels from which arise some important X-ray lines. The most important use of this gas is in the 'Neon lights' and fluorescent signs for advertisements. Neon contained in glow discharge lamps or high voltage discharge tubes at low pressure emits red light. In the presence of mercury vapors, the color of the glow turns blue. In daily life, most widespread use of Neon is in sodium vapour lamps for street lighting and in various pilot lamps for electronic equipments. In most types of fluorescent lights Neon is used in combination with other inert gases usually argon, krypton, and xenon. Neon is also used in scintillation counters, neutron fission counters, proportional counters, and ionization chambers for detection of charged particles. Its mixtures with bromine vapour and chlorine are used in Geiger tubes for counting nuclear particles. Helium-Neon mixture is used in gas lasers. Some other applications of Neon are in antifog devices, electrical current detectors, and lightning arrestors. The Neon gas is also used in welding and preparative reactions. In preparative reactions it provides an inert atmosphere to shield the reaction from air contact. Neon was discovered by Ramsay and Travers in 1898. Its name comes from the Greek word *neos*, which means new. It is present in the atmosphere at a concentration of 0.00182% by volume (dry atmosphere). This element is found in stars and interstellar gas clouds also. Earth's earliest crust probably contained Neon in minerals. Neon is derived commercially from the atmosphere. It is recovered from air after separation of oxygen and nitrogen in air separation plants.

Since 1921, when Ramsauer published his pioneer work on electron scattering from noble gases, there have been considerable interests in experimental and theoretical investigation on this subject due to its wide application discussed above. Due to development of high quality collimated electron and positron beam a lot of experimental measurements have been published but there is new possibility and scrutiny to do. They include differential and total cross sections and recently spin polarization cross sections and oscillator strength. Here we have summarized recent theoretical as well as experimental work focused on Neon.

In intermediate and high energy regions, the excitation of ground state of Neon by impact of electron is studied by so many researchers. Ballance and Griffin [2] have demonstrated a series of RMPS calculations of electron-impact excitation of Neon using recently developed parallel Breit–Pauli R-matrix program. In their calculations although the results clearly reveal the importance of coupling to the target continuum in Neon atom, the pseudo-state expansion is not yet sufficiently complete to provide reliable cross sections for energies above the ionization limit. Chen *et al* [3] have reported fully relativistic close-coupling calculation of the electron impact excitation of Neon using multiconfiguration Dirac-Fock (MCDF) and Dirac *R*-matrix method considering resonance and channel coupling effects. They demonstrated the strong resonances appeared in the excitation of the highly charged Neon in particular for intercombination and forbidden transitions. Comparing their results with experimental measurements of the integrated cross section at energies up to 400 eV and with other theoretical results, Srivastava *et al* [4] have used the relativistic distorted-wave approximation to calculate the excitation of the lowest metastable states of Neon and other inert atoms to the ten higher-lying fine-structure levels of the $np^5(n+1)p$ configuration. Their RDW calculations for the excitation of the metastable states of the noble gases yield that results are in generally good agreement with recent experimental results only at higher energies. At small projectile energies, Allan *et al* [5] have calculated absolute angle-differential cross sections for excitation of Neon atoms for $2p^5 3s$ and to selected $2p^5 3p$ levels as a function of electron energy up to 3.5 eV above threshold at the scattering angles of 0^0, 45^0, 90^0 , 135^0 and 180^0. In addition, the cross sections were reported as function of scattering angle from 0^0 to 180^0 at 18 eV for the $2p^5 3s$ levels and at 19.3 eV for the $2p^5 3p$ levels, respectively using the Breit–Pauli *B*-spline *R*-matrix method with non-orthogonal orbital sets. Recently Verma *et al* [6] have presented differential scattering cross section and total scattering cross section for the first excited state of Neon by electron as well as positron impact by choosing a complex type of potential, a part of which is directly calculated from the target charge density and other part is taken from Baluja and Jain [7]. A satisfactory comparison is found with different available theoretical and experimental data with their result. Zatsarinny and Bartshat [8] have reported large-scale *R*-matrix (close-coupling) with pseudostates calculations for electron scattering from Neon atoms in the nonrelativistic *LS*-coupling approximation with a recently developed parallel version of *B*-spline *R*-matrix codes. Their results confirm the very strong influence of coupling to the target continuum on theoretical predictions for excitation cross sections in Neon at intermediate energies previously reported by Ballance and Griffin. Zatsarinny and Bartschat [9] have reported results from a joint experimental and theoretical study of the angular momentum transfer in electron-impact excitation of the $(2p^6)\,^1S_0 \to (2p\,^53s)\,^1P_1$ resonance transition in Neon. Both the measured and calculated data show the circular light polarization P_3 to be positive for incident energy of 25 eV at scattering angles below 40^0. This observation implies a negative angular momentum transfer $L_\perp$.

Khakoo *et al* [10] have measured differential cross section measurements for the excitation of the $2p^53s$ configuration of Neon by using earlier data as calibration standards. They also present results from calculations of these differential cross sections using the *R*-matrix and unitarized first-order many-body theory, the distorted-wave Born approximation and relativistic distorted-wave methods. Comparison with available experimental differential cross sections and differential cross section ratios is also presented. In the energy range 16-19 eV, Bommels *et al* [11] have used an electron scattering apparatus combining a laser photoelectron source, a triply differentially pumped supersonic beam target, and several electron multipliers for simultaneous detection of elastically scattered electrons and of metastable atoms due to inelastic scattering for an improved study of electron-Neon scattering. Accurate values for the energies and widths of the low-lying Neon($2p^53s^2\,^2P_{3/2,1/2}$) Feshbach resonances have been determined from detailed analyses of the resonance profiles. The experimental data are also compared with theoretical results, calculated with an improved *R*-matrix approach. Very good overall agreement between the experimental and the theoretical results is observed. A very sharp Feshbach resonance, associated with the Neon $(2p^53p[5/2]_2)$ level, has been theoretically predicted and experimentally confirmed at 18.527 eV. Using magnetic angle changer and an electrostatic electron spectrometer, Linert *et al* [12] have reported differential cross sections for elastic electron scattering in Neon have been measured in the angular range of backward scattering from $110°–180°$ at incident energies of 7, 10, and 15eV. The differential cross sections measured in the above scattering angle range, together with results obtained previously in the range below 110°, have been integrated to obtain integral elastic and momentum transfer cross sections. Detailed comparison is presented of the measured differential and integral cross sections with the results of various theoretical calculations. With the use of magnetic angle-changing device Cho *et al* [13] have presented experimental and theoretical differential cross sections for the elastic scattering of electrons from Neon at four incident electron energies above the threshold from mid-angles to backward angles up to 180°. The results reveal some small differences between experiment and theory at backward angles in some cases. Matherson *et al* [14] have presented total absolute collision cross sections for Neon for ground state excitation using a recently developed experimental technique which utilizes a magneto-optical trap (MOT) and involves the measurement of MOT population dynamics to determine the cross section. Collision cross section measurements are presented for metastable Neon in the $^3P_2$ state. Jung *et al* [15] have presented experimental measurements for excitation cross sections into four $J=1$ levels of the $2p^53p$ configuration from $J=0$ and $J=2$ $2p^5$ 3s metastable levels. A complete set of cross sections into all ten levels of the $2p^53p$ configuration ($2p_x$ in Paschen's notation) from the ground state, the two metastable levels and the two resonance levels of the $2p^53s$ configuration ($1s_y$ in Paschen's notation) are compiled in convenient form. The resonance cross sections are obtained from an empirical scaling relationship between the measured metastable excitation cross sections and the corresponding optical oscillator strengths. Khakoo *et al* [16] have presented correction factors for DCS values of Neon after taking the observation by high resolution electron spectrometer and comparing the data by result of B-spline R-matrix method. In conclusion they suggest little modification in BSR method and TOF measurement.

3.2 THEORY

3.2.1 FOR ELASTIC SCATTERING

Elastic collisions of electrons with atoms are initiated as scattering of the projectile by the electrostatic field of the target atom. It is assumed that the atomic electron density $\rho(r)$ as a function of radius r, which is spherically symmetric; for atoms with open electron shells, this implies an average over orientations. Exchange between the projectile and the atomic electrons can be accounted for approximately by adding a local correction to the electrostatic interaction. In nonrelativistic (Schrodinger) theory, the wave function describing the scattering event is a distorted plane wave with the asymptotic form

$$\psi(r)_{r\to\infty} = \exp(i\,\boldsymbol{K}.\boldsymbol{r}) + \frac{\exp(iKr)}{r} f(\theta) \qquad\qquad \text{.... (3.1)}$$

where $\boldsymbol{r}$ is the position vector, $\boldsymbol{P} = \hbar\boldsymbol{k}$ is the momentum of the projectile, and $\hbar$ is the reduced Planck's constant. The differential cross section (DCS) for the scattering is completely determined by the scattering amplitude $f(\theta)$. In the relativistic formulation adopted here, $\psi(r)$ is a solution of the time-independent Dirac equation with the same potential. Dirac equations are

$$\frac{dP_l^{\pm}}{dr} = \frac{k^{\pm}}{r} P_l^{\pm}(r) + \frac{E-V+2mc^2}{c\,\hbar} Q_l^{\pm}(r) \qquad\qquad \text{.... (3.2a)}$$

$$\frac{dQ_l^{\pm}}{dr} = \frac{E-V}{c\,\hbar} P_l^{\pm}(r) + \frac{k^{\pm}}{r} Q_l^{\pm}(r) \qquad\qquad \text{.... (3.2b)}$$

where $P_l^{\pm}(r)$ and $Q_l^{\pm}(r)$ are radial wavefunctions. E is the kinetic energy of the projectile that is related to its total energy W by $E = W - mc^2$.

To calculate the DCS, the distorted wave [equation (3.1)] is expressed as a superposition of spherical waves (*i.e.,* eigenfunctions of the total angular momentum) that are computed numerically by solving the radial wave equation. In fact, phase shifts δ_l is required to determine the scattering amplitude and the DCS.

In the relativistic (Dirac) theory, the elastic-scattering differential cross section is expressed [17].

$$\frac{d\sigma_e}{d\Omega} = |f(\theta)|^2 + |g(\theta)|^2 \qquad \text{.... (3.3)}$$

Where $f(\theta)$ and $g(\theta)$ are the direct and spin-flip scattering amplitudes. These amplitudes are defined in terms of the phase shifts δ_l^+ and δ_l^- for spin-up and spin-down scattering, respectively.

$$f(\theta) = \frac{1}{2iK} \sum_l \{(l+1)[exp(2i\delta_l^+) - 1] + l[exp(2i\delta_l^-) - 1]\} P_l(cos\theta) \qquad \text{.... (3.4)}$$

$$g(\theta) = \frac{1}{2iK} \sum_l [exp(2i\delta_l^-) - exp(2i\delta_l^+)] P_l^1(cos\theta) \qquad \text{.... (3.5)}$$

In equation (3.4) and (3.5), $P_l(\theta)$ are the Legendre polynomials, and $P_l^1(\theta)$ are the associated Legendre polynomials.

The phase shifts δ_l^+ are obtained from the large r behavior of radial wavefunctions, $P_l^\pm(r)$ and $Q_l^\pm(r)$, which are calculated by integrating the radial Dirac equations (3.2-a,b). Using Buhring's power series method [18] based on a cubic-spline interpolation of the potential function, $rV(r)$ is expressed as a piecewise cubic polynomial in r

$$r V(r) = a_n + b_n r + c_n r^2 + d_n r^3 \qquad \text{.... (3.6)}$$

With the condition

$$r_1 = 0 < r_2 \ldots \ldots \ldots < r_{N-1} < r_N \qquad \text{.... (3.7)}$$

In the interval $(r_n < r_{n+1})$, the radial functions can be formally expressed by the power series

$$P_l^\pm(r) = r^\alpha \sum_{i=0}^{\infty} P_i r^i \qquad \text{and}$$

$$Q_l^\pm(r) = r^\beta \sum_{i=0}^{\infty} Q_i r^i \qquad \text{.... (3.8)}$$

Salvat and Mayol [19] have given method of solving the coefficients by values of $P_l^\pm(r_n)$ and $Q_l^\pm(r_n)$ at the end point of the interval.

The interaction potential (Dirac-Hartree-Fock potential) is defined as

$$V(r) = -e\,\varphi(r) + V_{exc}(r) \qquad\qquad \text{.... (3.9)}$$

where $\varphi(r)$ is the electrostatic potential of the target atom.

$$\varphi(r) = \frac{Ze}{r} - e\left(\frac{1}{r}\int_0^r \rho(r')\,4\pi r'^2 dr' + \int_0^\infty \rho(r')\,4\pi r'\,dr'\right) \qquad \text{.... (3.10)}$$

$\rho(r)$ is the atomic electron density. The term $V_{exc}(r)$ in equation (3.9) is a local approximation to the exchange interaction between the projectile and the electrons in the target. Furness and McCarthy [20] have given the exchange potential as

$$V_{exc}(r) = \frac{1}{2}[E + e\varphi(r)] - \frac{1}{2}\left\{[E + e\varphi(r)]^2 + 4\pi\frac{\hbar^2 e^2}{m}\right\}^{\frac{2}{}} \qquad \text{..... (3.11)}$$

Thus interaction potential is completely determined by atomic density $\rho(r)$.

The integration of the radial equations is started from $r = 0$ with boundary values

$$P_l^\pm(0) = 0 \text{ , and } Q_l^\pm(0) = 0 \qquad\qquad \text{.... (3.12)}$$

In the first interval from $r_1 = 0$ to r_2 [equation (3.7)], the constants α and β are different from zero and are determined by the angular momentum quantum numbers as Salvat and Moyal [19].

After determining the values of the radial wavefunction at r_2, the solution is extended outwards by using series expansions equation (3.8) (with $\alpha = \beta = 0$) upto certain radial distance , r_{max} , large enough to ensure that the potential energy of the electron $V(r)$ is neglible as compared to its kinetic energy.

At sufficiently large distance r, the radial function $P_l^\pm(r)$ adopts the asymptotic form

$$P_l^\pm(r) \cong \sin\left(Kr - l\frac{\pi}{2} + \delta_l^\pm\right) \qquad\qquad \text{.... (3.13)}$$

Where $\hbar K = \dfrac{1}{c}\sqrt{E(E + 2mc^2)}$ $\qquad\qquad$ .... (3.14)

is the momentum of the projectile . Equation (3.13), which confers a geometrical meaning to the phase shift, is not directly usable to compute $\delta_l^{\pm}$ because $P_l^{\pm}(r)$ reaches the form given by equation (3.13) only at a distance r that may be much larger than r_{max}. Instead, the phase shift is obtained from the calculated values of radial function at r_{max} by matching the numerical solution to the exact solution for $r > r_{max}$ $(V = 0)$ that can be expressed as a linear combination of spherical Bessel functions $j_k(Kr)$ and $n_k(Kr)$ with indices $k = l, l \pm 1$ as in [21].

3.2.2 FOR INELASTIC SCATTERING

We have considered the distorted wave Born approximation (DWBA) theory for electron impact excitation of atoms. Suppose an incident electron of momentum $\mathbf{k}_i$ collides with an atom A, after the collision, the scattered electron has momentum $\mathbf{k}_f$, and one bound electron in atom A is excited to a higher energy bound state. In the frozen core approximation, the 'exact' Hamiltonian for the whole system is

$$H = -\frac{1}{2}\nabla_1^2 + V_{A^+}(\mathbf{r}_1) - \frac{1}{2}\nabla_2^2 + V_{A^+}(\mathbf{r}_2) + \frac{1}{r_{12}} \qquad \ldots\ldots (3.15)$$

where $\mathbf{r}_1$ and $\mathbf{r}_2$ are the position vectors for the projectile and the bound state electron with respect to the nucleus, respectively. This Hamiltonian can be rewritten approximately as

$$H_j = -\frac{1}{2}\nabla_1^2 + U_j(\mathbf{r}_1) - \frac{1}{2}\nabla_2^2 + V_{A^+}(\mathbf{r}_2) \qquad (j = i, f). \qquad .... (3.16)$$

In this equation, $U_i(U_f)$ is the distorting potential used to calculate the initial (final) state wavefunction $\chi_{\mathbf{k}_i}\left(\chi_{\mathbf{k}_f}\right)$ for the projectile. In the DWBA, the direct transition amplitude for excitation from an initial state ψ_i to a final state ψ_f can be expressed as

$$f = \langle \chi_{\mathbf{k}_f}^{-}(1)\psi_f(2)|V_i|\psi_i(2)\chi_{\mathbf{k}_i}^{-}(1)\rangle, \qquad .... (3.17)$$

where V_i is the perturbation interaction:

$$V_i = H - H_i = \frac{1}{r_{12}} + V_{A^+}(\mathbf{r}_1) - U_i(\mathbf{r}_1) \qquad \text{.... (3.18)}$$

In equation (3.17), the initial and final state wavefunctions for the projectile satisfy the differential equation

$$\left[-\frac{1}{2}\nabla_1^2 + U_j(\mathbf{r}_1) - \frac{1}{2}k_j^2\right]\chi_{\mathbf{k}_j}(\mathbf{r}_1) = 0 \quad (j = i, f) \qquad \text{.... (3.19)}$$

and the bound state wavefunctions are the eigenfunctions of the equation

$$\left[-\frac{1}{2}\nabla_2^2 + V_{A^+}(\mathbf{r}_2) - \epsilon_j\right]\psi_j(\mathbf{r}_2) = 0 \quad (j = i, f) \qquad \text{.... (3.20)}$$

where $\epsilon_j (j = i, f)$ are the corresponding eigenenergies of the initial and final bound states which can be expressed as

$$\psi_j(r) = \psi_{N_j L_j} Y_{L_j M_j}(\hat{\mathbf{r}}) \quad (j = i, f) \qquad \text{.... (3.21)}$$

The exchange scattering amplitude is given by

$$g = \langle\psi_f(1)\rangle\chi_{\mathbf{k}_f}^-(2)|V_i|\psi_i(2)\chi_{\mathbf{k}_i}^+(1) \qquad \text{.... (3.22)}$$

Finally, the differential cross section for electron impact excitation is given by

$$\frac{d\sigma}{d\Omega} = N(2\pi)^4 \frac{k_f}{k_i} \frac{1}{2L_i+1} \times \sum_{M_i=-L_i}^{+L_i} \sum_{M_f=-L_f}^{+L_f} \left(\frac{3}{4}|f - g|^2 + \frac{1}{4}|f + g|^2\right)$$

$$\text{.... (3.23)}$$

The prefactor N in equation (3.23) denotes the number of electrons in the subshell from which one electron is excited.

The distorting potentials, U_i and U_f, used in equation (3.19) to calculate the wavefunctions for the projectile in the initial and final states, respectively, are not determined directly by the formalism. Here, we use static potentials which take the form as

$$U_j\,(r_1) = V_{A^+}(r_1) + \int dr_2 \frac{|\psi_j(\mathbf{r_2})|^2}{r_{12}} \qquad (j = i, f) \qquad \qquad \dots (3.24)$$

$V_{A^+}(r)$ in equation (3.24) is the atomic potential used to evaluate eigenstate wavefunctions of the bound state electron. Here we take the effective potential from Tong and Lin [22] based on single active electron approximation, which is given by

$$V_{A^+}(r) = -\frac{1 + a_1 e^{-a_2 r} + a_3 r\, e^{-a_4 r} + a_5 e^{-a_6 r}}{r} \qquad \qquad \dots (3.25)$$

where the parameters a_i , as given explicitly in table 1 in [22], are obtained by fitting the calculated binding energies from this potential to the experimental ones of the ground state and the first few excited states of the target atom.

3.3   RESULT AND DISCUSSION

We have calculated elastic differential cross section (DCS) for Neon by electron impact using equation (3.3) at 100 eV and 300 eV which is outcome of solutions of radial Dirac equations (3.2a,3.2b). In determination of related phase shift, we have used Dirac-Hartree-Fock (DHF) type potential. Also, we have computed inelastic scattering cross section of 3s, 3p, 4s and 4p configurations of Neon for incident energies 30 and 50 eV. In inelastic scattering cross section we have used distorted wave Born approximation (DWBA) as equation (3.23). Our results along with other available experimental results are plotted in figures (3.1) and (3.2) for elastic scattering whereas figures (3.3) to (3.10) for inelastic scattering.

3.3.1   ELASTIC SCATTERING

Figure (3.1) shows our result of elastic scattering cross section of Neon by electron impact at 100 eV. For comparison we have plotted experimental results (E) of Gupta and Rees [23]. From figure it is seen that our results are in agreement with experimental data. However, the magnitude of DCS is little smaller than the experimental result with same position of minima.

Figure (3.2) shows our results of elastic scattering cross section of Neon by electron impact at 30 eV along with experimental result (E) of Gupta and Rees [23]. It is seen that the present results are in very good agreement between scattering angle 25^0 to 90^0. However our results slightly differ with experimental data in smaller and higher angular range both. At this impact energy no minima is observed.

3.3.2 INELASTIC SCATTERING

3s – Excitation

Figure (3.3) gives the plot of inelastic differential scattering cross section of 3s state of Neon at incident electron energy 30 eV. For comparison we have plotted experimental measurements (R) of Register *et al* [24]. Up to 60^0, our result is in good agreement with the experimental result. Then after a little discrepancy can be observed till the last available experimental data but nature of variation of both the curves is still same.

Figure (3.4) is the same as figure (3.3) but at the incident energy 50 eV. At this energy our result is in excellent agreement with available experimental data of Register *et al* [24]. However, no data is available after scattering angle 125^0.

3p – Excitation

Figures (3.5) and (3.6) show our results of inelastic scattering cross section of 3p state of Neon at incident electron energy 30 and 50 eV respectively. Here again the experimental data (R) of Register *et al* [24] is plotted for the comparison purpose. From figure, we noticed that both the results are comparable in the lower angular region $(\theta < 30^0)$. However in large angular region, our results tend to overestimate the experimental results showing the position of secondary minima almost same in both figures. It is difficult to comment on present results in higher angular range as no data is available at both energies.

4s – Excitation

Figures (3.7) and (3.8) show the variation of the differential scattering cross sections for 4s state of Neon at incident electron energy 30 and 50 eV respectively. The same experimental results of Register *et al* [24] are plotted in both the figures. It is clearly seen that below 60^0, the present results show a nice agreement with data. However at 30 eV impact energy the experimental data left smoothness and shows irregularity in the magnitude of DCS. The present result shows a smooth and almost constant variation in DCS. If we increase impact energy, both present and experimental result almost reproduce each other. It is an encouraging feature at this impact energy.

4p – Excitation

Figures (3.9) and (3.10) show the angular variation of the differential scattering cross sections for 4p state of Neon at incident electron energy 30 and 50 eV respectively. The same comparison is plotted in both the figures as we did in earlier figure. It can be seen in figure (3.9) that the present results differ in very small magnitude with experimental results up to 120^0. But as scattering angle increases the gap between present result and experimental data also increases. In figure (3.10) below 40^0 angles the present results are in excellent agreement with data. A remarkable difference can be observed as scattering angle increases.

3.4   CONCLUDING REMARKS

In conclusion we purpose that more theoretical calculations are required for Neon elastic scattering as well as inelastic scattering, as we have already described in introduction part of this chapter that Neon atom is most important inert atom in various field of science and technology. Theoretically our approach is simpler approach whose computational part can be performed very easily. This method can also be modified by including the relativistic calculations.

<u>FIGURE CAPTIONS</u>

Figure [3.1]   **: DCS for elastic scattering of Neon by impact of electron at 100 eV**

——————   : Present result

● ● ● ●   : Experimental result of Gupta and Rees [23]

Figure [3.2]   **: DCS for elastic scattering of Neon by impact of electron at 300 eV**

——————   : Present result

● ● ● ●   : Experimental result of Gupta and Rees [23]

Figure [3.3]   **: DCS for 3s excitation of Neon by impact of electron at 30 eV**

——————   : Present result

● ● ● ●   : Experimental result of Register *et al* [24]

Figure [3.4]   **: DCS for 3s excitation of Neon by impact of electron at 50 eV**

——————   : Present result

● ● ● ●   : Experimental result of Register *et al* [24]

Figure [3.5]   **: DCS for 3p excitation of Neon by impact of electron at 30 eV**

——————   : Present result

● ● ● ●   : Experimental result of Register *et al* [24]

DCS FOR ELASTIC SCATTERING OF NEON BY IMPACT OF ELECTRON AT 100 eV

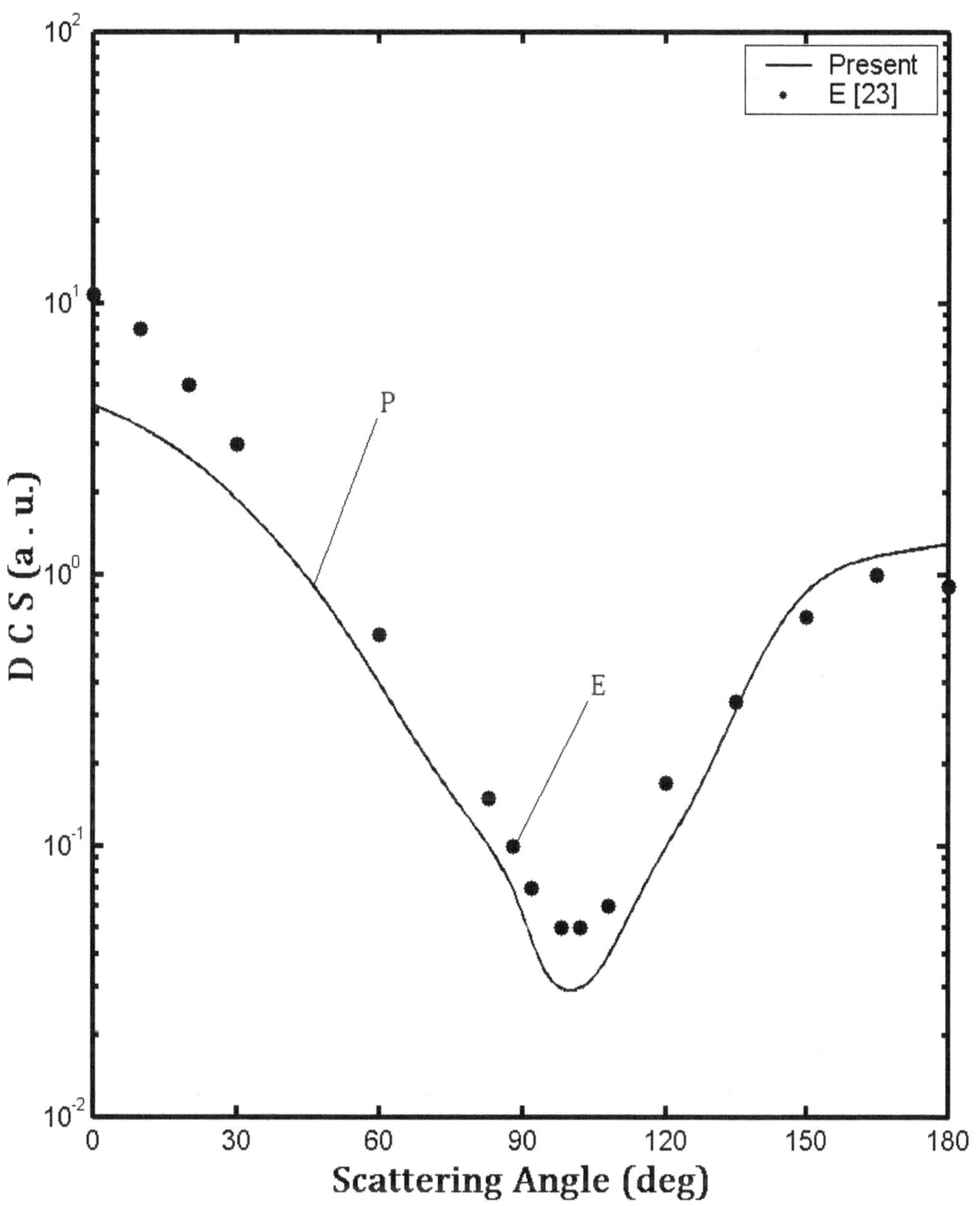

FIGURE [3.1]

DCS FOR ELASTIC SCATTERING OF NEON BY IMPACT OF ELECTRON AT 300 eV

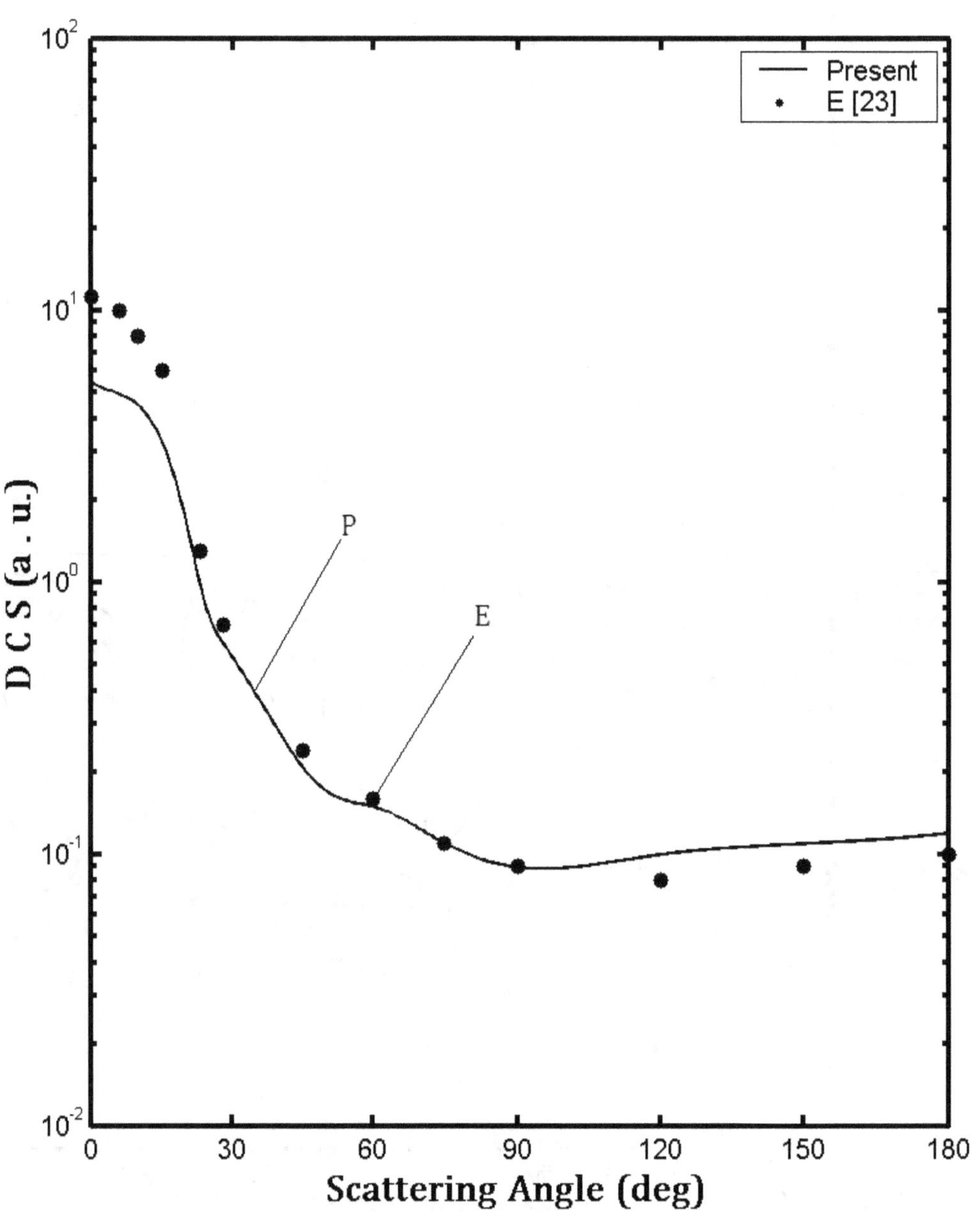

FIGURE [3.2]

DCS FOR (3s) EXCITATION OF NEON BY IMPACT OF ELECTRON AT 30 eV

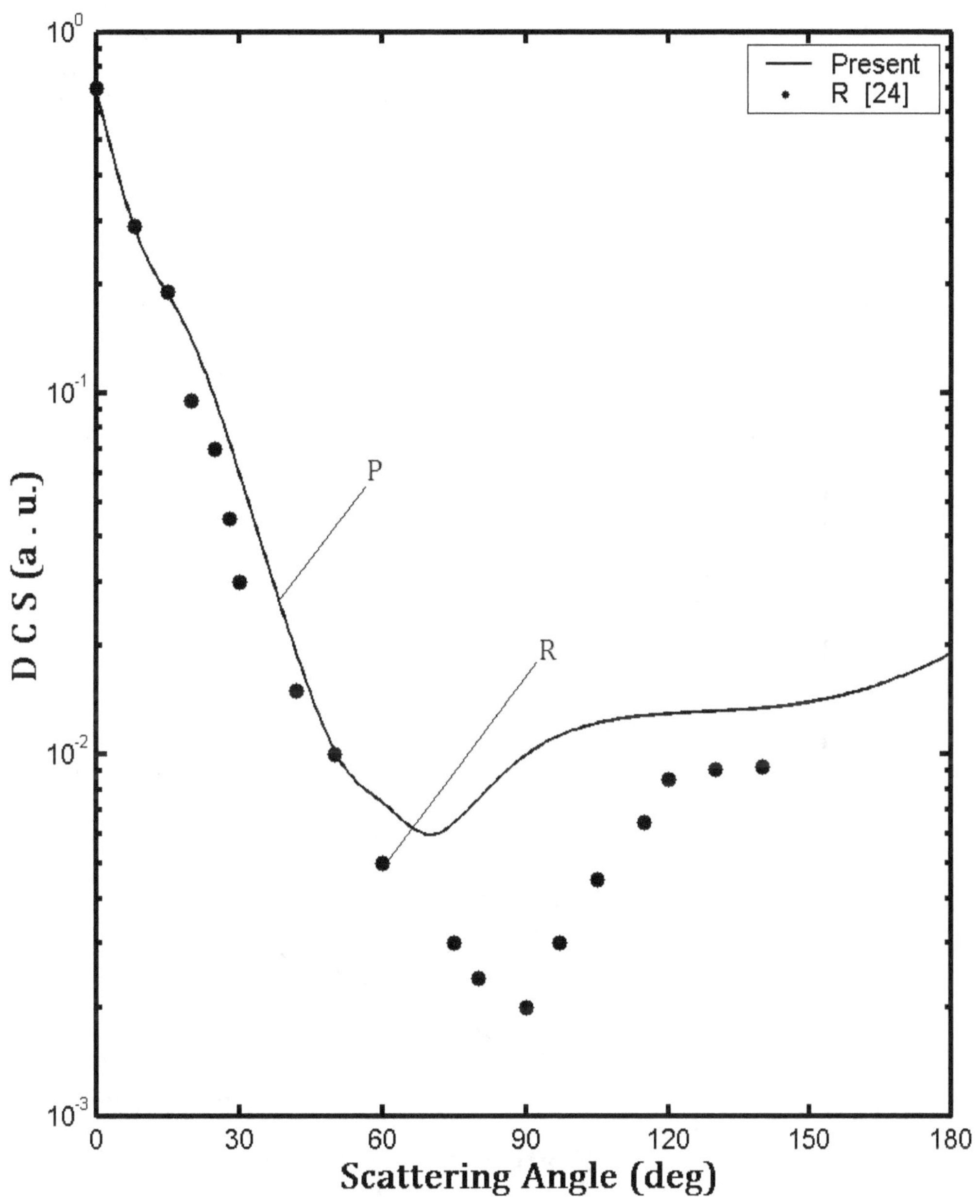

FIGURE [3.3]

DCS FOR (3s) EXCITATION OF NEON BY IMPACT OF ELECTRON AT 50 eV

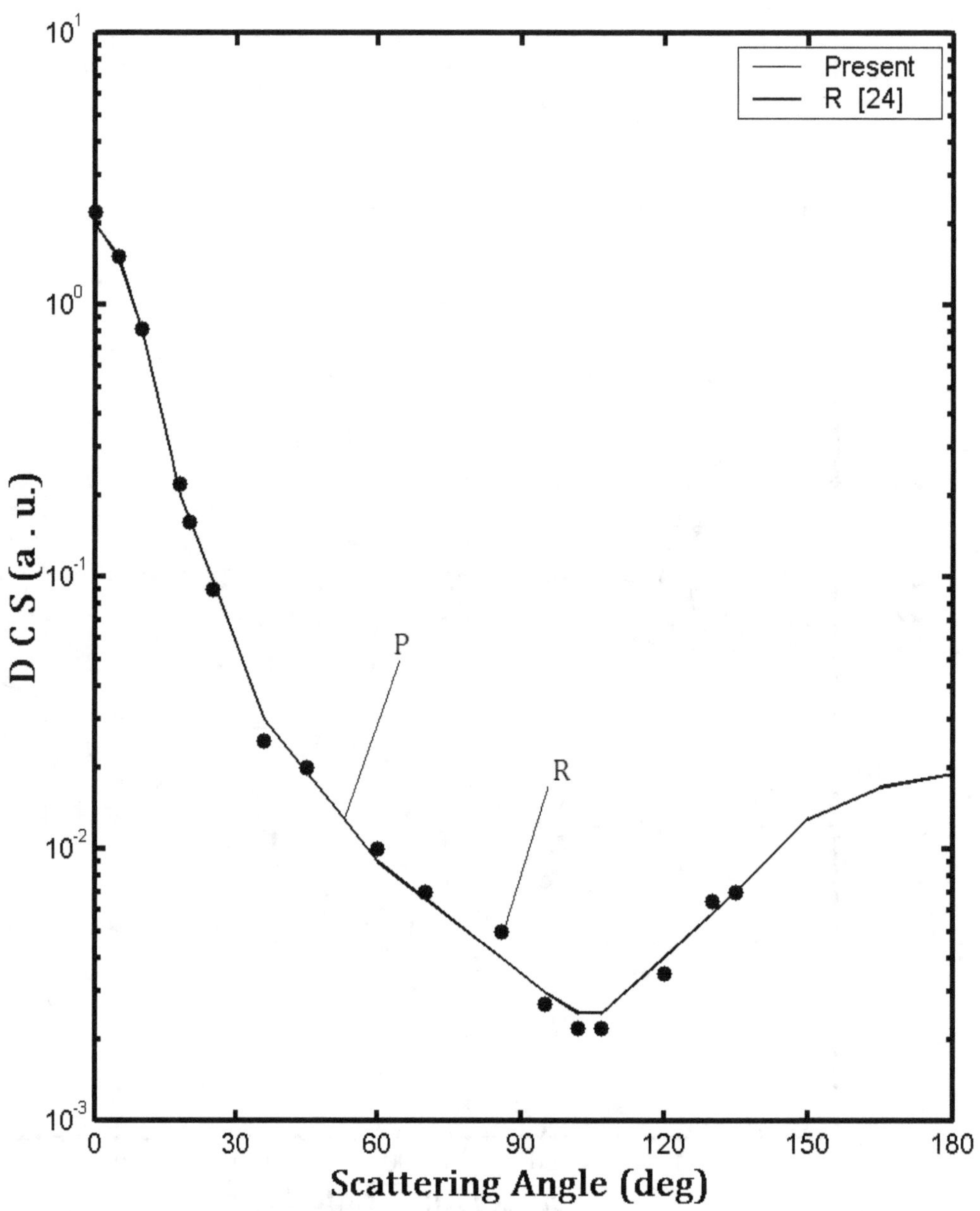

FIGURE [3.4]

DCS FOR (3p) EXCITATION OF NEON BY

IMPACT OF ELECTRON AT 30 eV

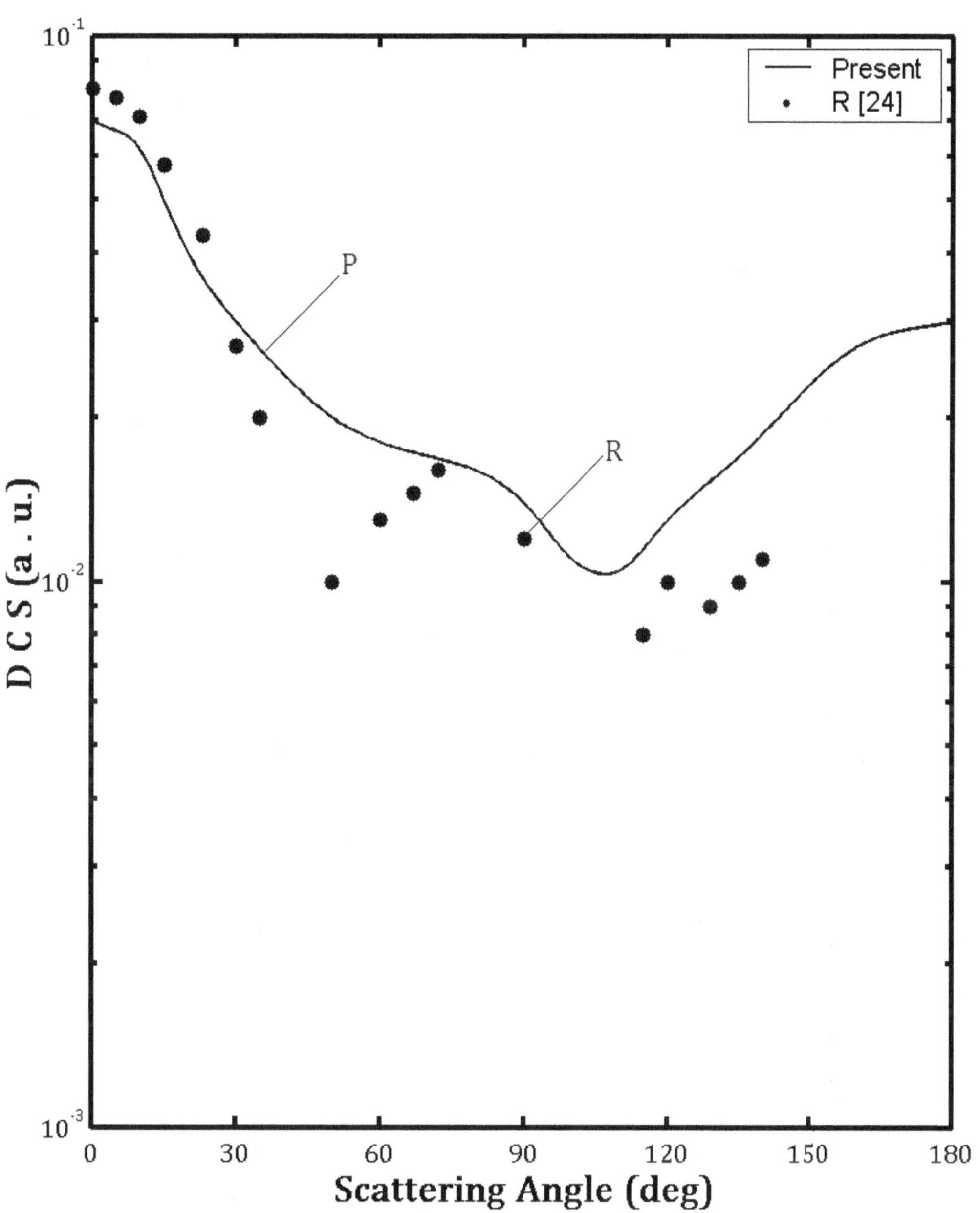

FIGURE [3.5]

DCS FOR (3p) EXCITATION OF NEON BY IMPACT OF ELECTRON AT 50 eV

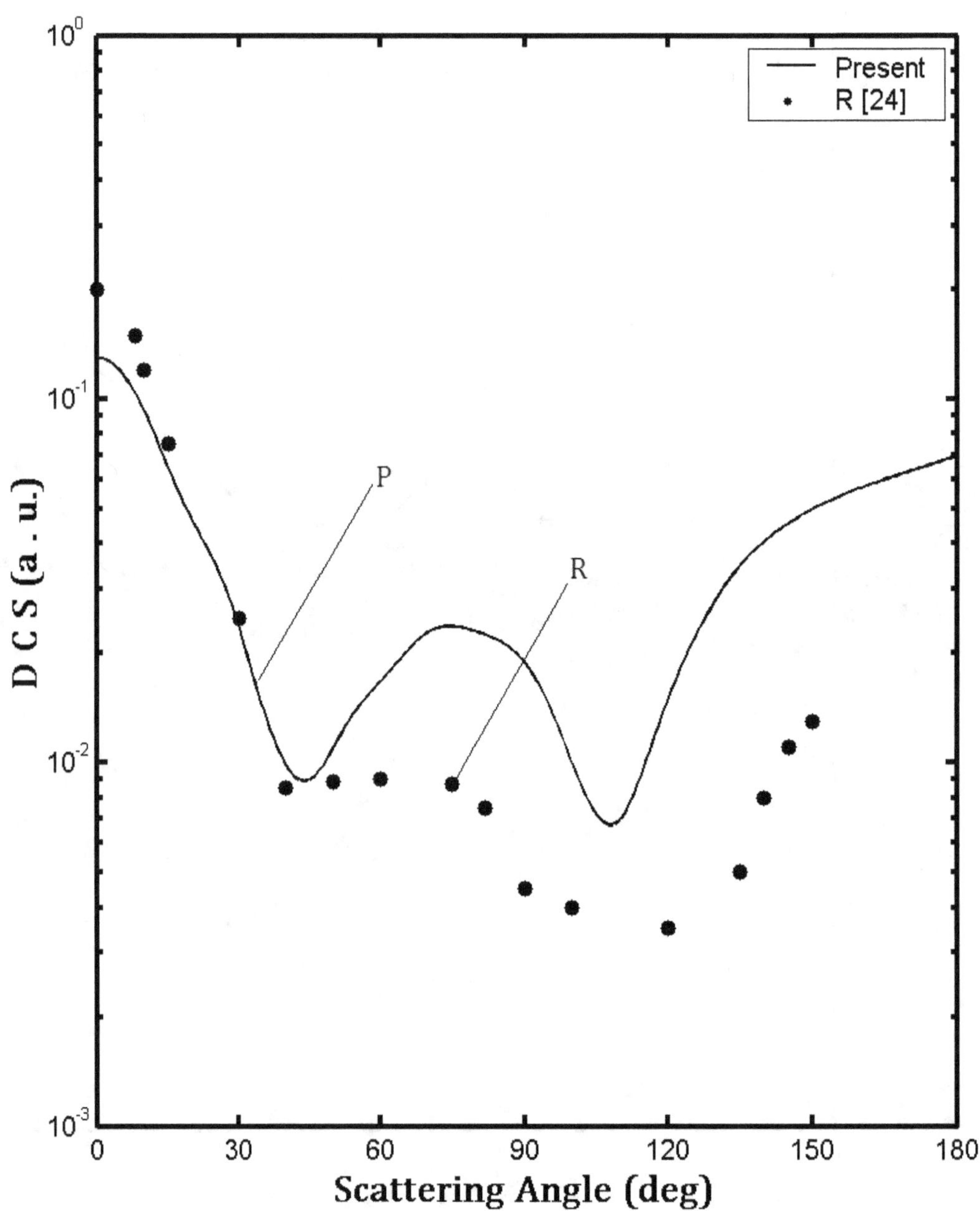

FIGURE [3.6]

DCS FOR (4s) EXCITATION OF NEON BY IMPACT OF ELECTRON AT 30 eV

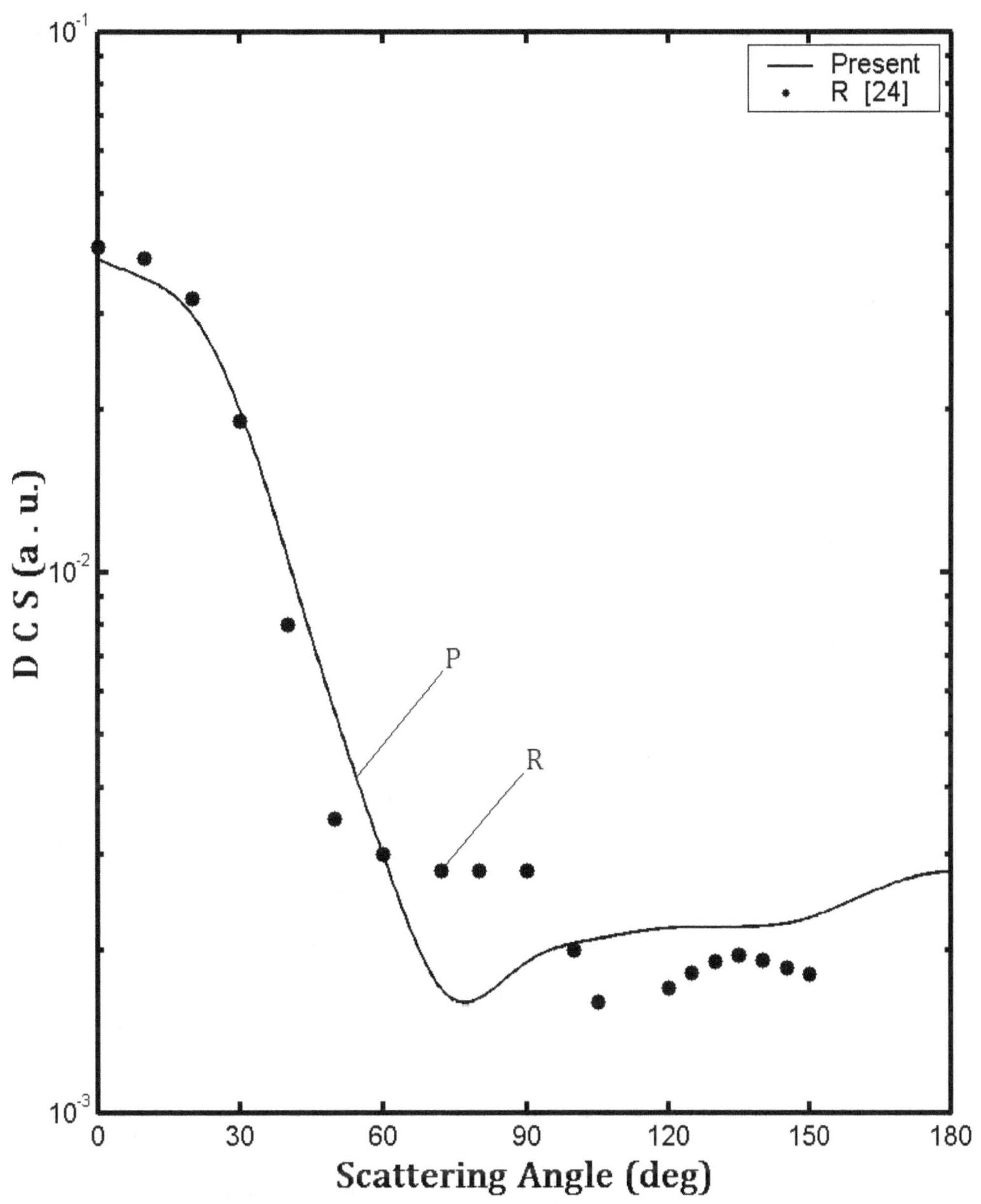

FIGURE [3.7]

DCS FOR (4s) EXCITATION OF NEON BY IMPACT OF ELECTRON AT 50 eV

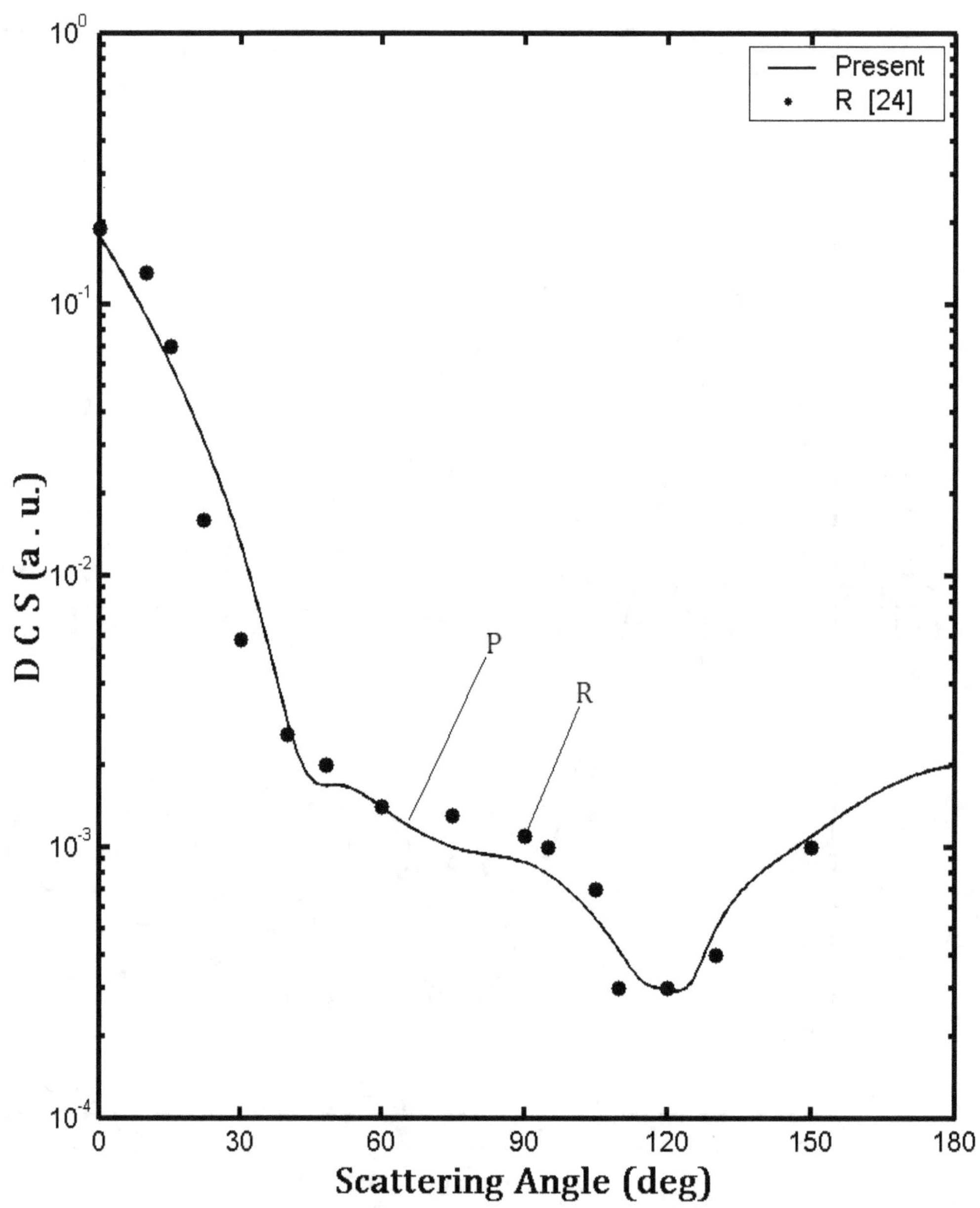

FIGURE [3.8]

DCS FOR (4p) EXCITATION OF NEON BY

IMPACT OF ELECTRON AT 30 eV

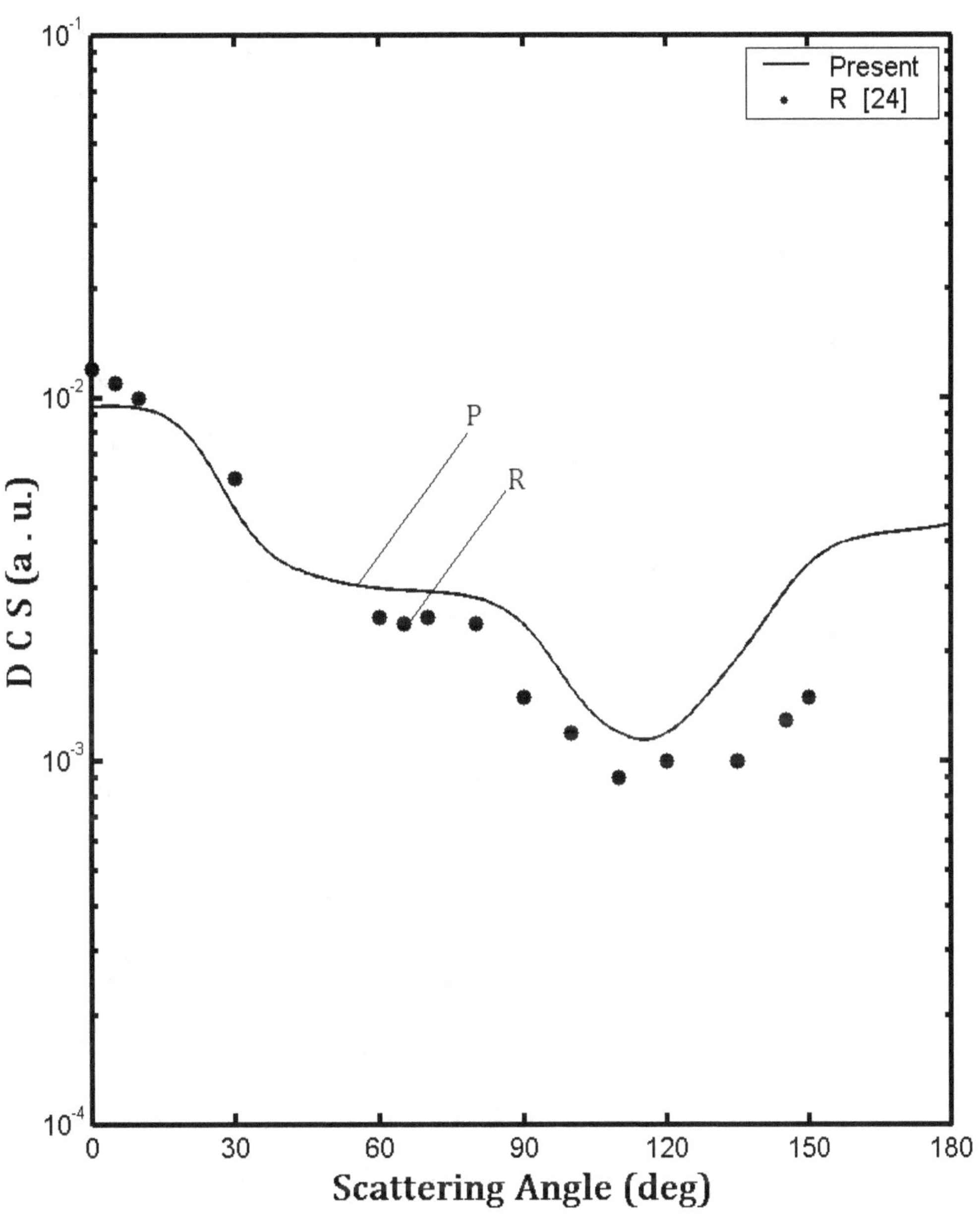

FIGURE [3.9]

DCS FOR (4p) EXCITATION OF NEON BY IMPACT OF ELECTRON AT 50 eV

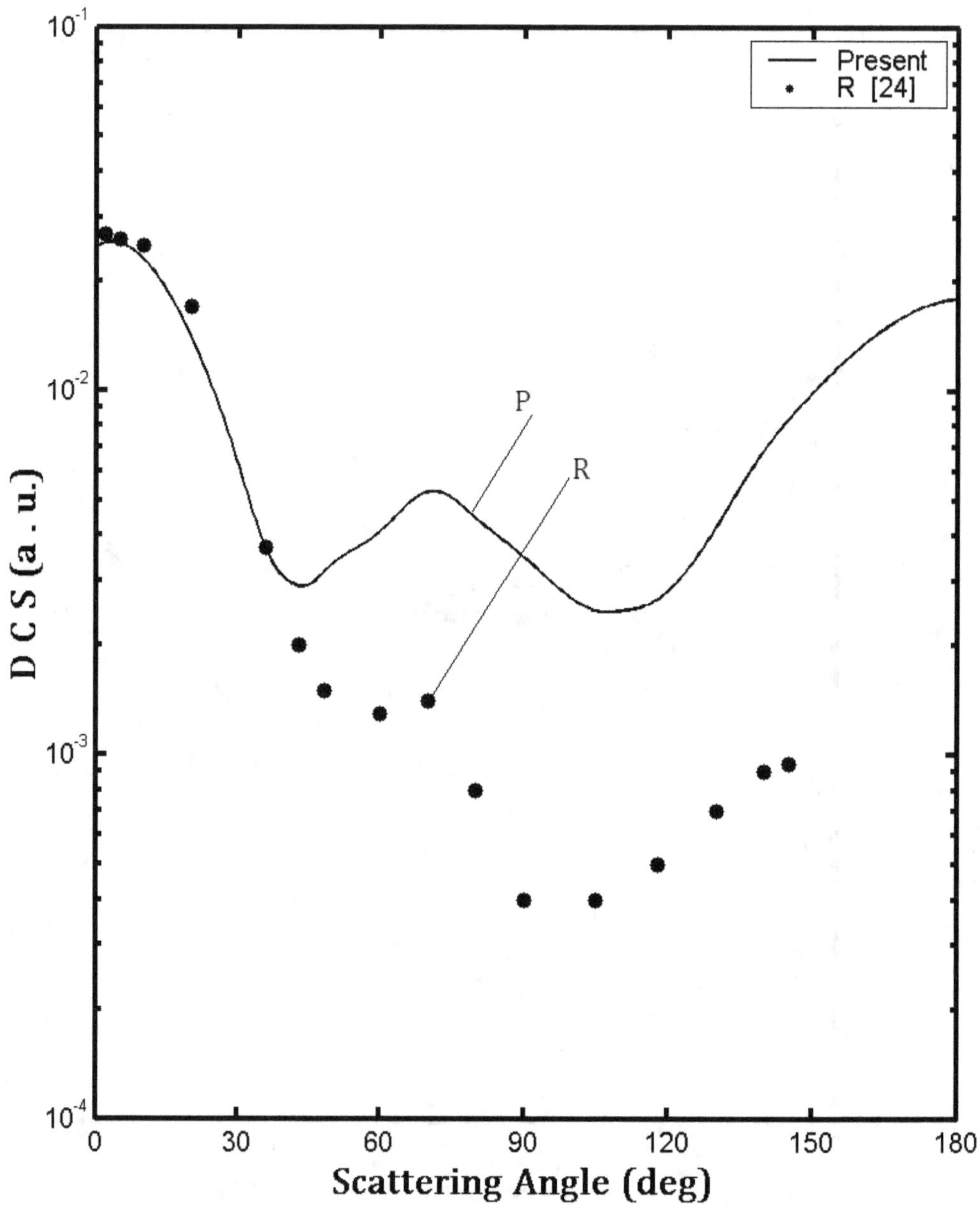

FIGURE [3.10]

REFERENCES

1.   S. J. Buckman and C.W. Clark, Rev. Mod. Phys. **66**, 539 (1994).

2.   C. P. Ballance and D. C. Griffin, *J. Phys. B: At. Mol. Opt. Phys.* **37**, 2943 (2004).

3.   G. X. Chen, R. K. Smith, K. Kirby, N. S. Brickhouse, and B. J. Wargelin, Phys. Rev. A **74**, 042709 (2006).

4.   Rajesh Srivastava, A. D. Stauffer, and Lalita Sharma, Phy. Rev. A **74**, 012715 (2006).

5.   M. Allan, K. Franz, H. Hotop, O. Zatsarinny and K. Bartschat, J. Phys. B: At. Mol. Opt. Phys. **42**, 044009 (2009) .

6.   K. R. Verma, K. K. Sharma and S. Saxena, *Recent Research in Science & Technology* **3**(**6**), 91-94 (2011).

7.   K. L. Baluja and A. Jain, Phys. Rev A, **46**, 1279 (1992) .

8.   O. Zatsarinny and K. Bartschat, Phys. Rev. A **85**, 062710 (2012).

9.   O. Zatsarinny and K. Bartschat, Phys. Rev. A **85**, 050701(R) (2012).

10.   M. A. Khakoo *et al*, Phys. Rev. A **65**, 062711 (2002).

11.   J. Bommels, K. Franz, T. H. Hoffmann, A. Gopalan, O. Zatsarinny, K. Bartschat, M. W. Ruf, and H. Hotop, Phys. Rev. A **71**, 012704 (2005).

12.   I. Linert, B.Mielewska, George C. King, and M. Zubek, Phys. Rev. A **74**, 042701 (2006).

13.   H. Cho, H. Tanaka, R. P. McEachran and S. J. Buckman, Phys. Rev. A 78, 034702 (2008).

14.   K. J. Matherson, R. D. Glover, D. E. Laban, and R. T. Sang, Phys. Rev. A **78**, 042712 (2008).

15.   R. O. Jung, Garrett A. Piech, M. L. Keeler, J. B. Boffard, L. W. Anderson, and C. Lin, J. Appl. Phys. **109**, 123303 (2011).

16.   M. A. Khakoo, O. Zatsarinny and K. Bartschat, J. Phys. B: At. Mol. Opt. Phys. **44** 085201 (2011).

17.   D. W. Walker, Adv. Phys. **20**, 257(1971).

18.   W. Buhring, Z. Phys. **187**, 180 (1965).

19.   F. Salvat and R. Moyal, Comput. Phys. Commun. **74**, 358(1991).

20.   J. B. Furness and I. E. McCathy, J. Phys. B:At. Mol. Phys. **6**, 2280 (1973).

21.   L. H. Thomas, J. Chem. Phys. **22**, 1758(1954).

22.   X. M. Tong and C.D. Lin, J. Phys. B: At. Mol. Opt. Phys. **38**, 2593(2005).

23.   S. C. Gupta and J. A. Rees, J. Phys. B: At. Mol. Phys. **8**, 417 (1975).

24.   D.F. Register, S. Trajmar, G. Steffensen and D. C. Cartwright, Phys. Rev. A **29**, 1793 (1984).

CHAPTER-4

SCATTERING OF ELECTRON AND POSITRON FROM ARGON

4.1 INTRODUCTION

The study of atomic collision provides the most energetic means available to physicists for understanding various branches of science and advance technology. The comparative study of electron and positron yields the useful information about different interaction potentials at work in collision dynamics. The accurate determination of scattering parameters and understanding of electron/positron impact atomic collision processes is important for a number of reasons. From a practical perspective, the modeling of many systems of environmental and technological interest relies on the incorporation of cross section data to describe collision processes at the microscopic scale. These cross sections predict reaction rates for the range of possible collision outcomes comprising elastic scattering, excitation, ionization and polarization *etc*. Thus the provision of precise cross-section data plays a vital role to these applications. Sometimes, particularly in scattering and excitation from the ground state, cross sections can be calculated more accurately than they can presumably be measured. Also, on the other hand, measurements involving optically unstable initial states can be very difficult and are often impossible with currently available experimental techniques. Experimental benchmark data, therefore, may provide a crucial touchstone to both assess and to drive new developments in atomic collision theory and enhance its predictive powers. From a broader perspective, studies of electron-atom collisions contribute to our understanding of the electronic structure of matter by providing a well defined testing ground to explore the behavior of many-electron systems. In the area of electron-atom collisions, the electron/positron-noble gas systems have been a prime focus of study over many years. These non reactive gases can be easily handled and do not contaminate sensitive apparatus. As a consequence, they are particularly conducive to the measurement of accurate cross section data, which can assist in the development of theory for all atomic species, including those whose reactivity renders experiments infeasible.

The scattering of positrons by atoms is very different from the corresponding electron atom scattering. Apparently it may be seen that only a charge of sign in the interaction potential is involved. In the presence of a projectile, the atomic cloud is distorted. It is interesting to note that the effect of distortion of the atom is attractive in nature for both cases. The importance of the polarization potential in low energy electron-atom scattering processes is well known. For electrons, the potential due to polarization tends to add to the static potential which, being attractive tends to cancel the static interaction which is repulsive. These differences provide useful information in assessing the relative importance of the polarization potential. At low incident positron energies the effect of polarization is found to be large enough to cause the positron to be, on the whole, attracted to the atom. The interaction of a low-energy positron with a many-electron atom is characterized by strong correlation effects. Apart from the dynamic polarization of the electron cloud by the field of the positron, the positron can also form positronium (Ps), by picking up one of the atomic electrons. When the positron energy is below the Ps-formation threshold, $\varepsilon_{Ps} = I + E_{1s}(Ps) = I - 6.8 eV$ where I is the atomic ionization potential, positronium formation is a virtual process. Another fundamental difference between positron and electron scattering is that the positron, unlike the electron, is distinguishable from the target electrons. In the case of electron scattering, the nature of the total wave function is fully guided by Pauli's principle, whereas in the positron scattering case, our knowledge of the total wave function is incomplete for small separations. In common with electron-atom collisions, many processes can occur during the interaction of positrons with atoms. At low energies, elastic scattering is usually the only open channel apart from annihilation which has a relatively negligible effect compared with any other processes. As the incident positron energy increases, various inelastic channels become accessible, including positronium formation, target excitation and ionization. For positron-helium collisions, for example, the elastic scattering remains the only open channel for energies below the Ps formation threshold of 17.8 eV [1]. During the last 20 years positron-atom collision problems have been studied extensively. The development of new experimental techniques to obtain low energy monoenergetic beam has stimulated this surge of activity [2]. A comprehensive review of progress in the positron-atom (molecule) scattering has been given by many researchers. In spite of the important advances in recent years, both theoretically and experimentally, our knowledge of positron-atom scattering is still incomplete. The change of the sign of the charge in positron-atom scattering as opposed to the electron-atom scattering has several important consequences. The exchange effects between the projectile and the target electrons are absent. In contrast to the electron, the positron is attracted by the target electrons and repelled by the nuclei. This attraction must be taken into account adequately if accurate results are to be obtained. In the case of positron scattering by atoms the static potential energy is positive, whereas the lowest order term in the polarization potential is negative. Thus two major components in the positron-target interaction tend to cancel each other. The slow positron scattering has the specificity that the incident positron combines with one of the electrons in the target to produce a bound positron-electron system (positronium). That is to say, a new inelastic threshold appears where positronium formation is energetically allowed. This inelastic threshold always lies below the first inelastic threshold of excitation. The theoretical analysis of positron scattering from atomic systems represents a very difficult task of scattering theory, require that a double perturbative expansion, with respect to both positron electron and electron-electron Coulomb interactions, respectively, be carried out. In the case of positron Helium scattering, better results have been obtained by the variational methods [2-4], and the optical potential method [5- 8].

Argon has been a favorite scattering target for both experimentalists and theorists as most ubiquitous noble gas of the earth's atmosphere. Its closed outer shell means simple to describe theoretically and non-reactivity makes it easy to handle experimentally. Electron-impact excitation of neutral Argon is of both fundamental and applied interest. It has been studied theoretically and experimentally for many years and excitation data for Argon are of significant importance to the modeling of a variety of laboratory plasmas and other lighting applications discussed later. Argon has relatively high excitation threshold leading to a large energy interval where elastic scattering is the only open channel. In this region, the scattering of electrons and positrons from these gases can be well described by a potential scattering model containing the static and polarization interactions between the incident particle and the target plus exchange in the case of electrons. Argon gas has been studied from the discharge point of view for more than 100 years and interest in this gas is due to several important fundamental and technical considerations. Its presence in high concentrations plays a major role in the performance of the high pressure laser system and in direct nuclear-pumped lasing media.

Argon was discovered by Lord Raleigh and Sir William Ramsay in 1894. It is the third most abundant element in the atmosphere. Its concentration in air is 0.934% by volume. Also, it occurs in earth's crust at a concentration of 3.4 mg/kg, and in the sea water at 4.3 µg/L. Ar-40 has been detected in the atmosphere of Mars, estimated to be about 1.6% by volume. Argon has numerous applications in metallurgy, cryogenic, electronic, laboratory and as light sources. It is used in low pressure gas discharge tubes as a filler gas, emitting bluish light. It is also used in mercury and sodium-vapor lamps mixed with other inert gases. In metallurgy it is used to shield and protect welding metal arcs; in surface cleaning of metals; as a working fluid in plasma arc devices; as an inert blanket in melting and casting of certain alloys; to atomize molten metals and produce their powder; and in high temperature soldering and refining operations; and powder metal sintering. In the laboratory, Argon is used as a carrier gas in gas chromatography; or for metal analysis by furnace atomic absorption or inductively coupled plasma emission spectrophotometry; and as a filler gas (often mixed with other gas) in Geiger–Muller, proportional cosmic ray and scintillation counters. It is also used as inert atmosphere in glove boxes to carry out reactions and handling of air-sensitive substances. Argon is used as a low-temperature cryogenic fluid for isothermal baths. It is also used in air sampling by condensing the air in a trap and subsequently analyzing organic pollutants. In electronic industry Argon and helium are used as protective atmosphere and heat-transfer medium to grow single crystals of ultrapure semiconductors; and as diluents and carriers of dopant gases such as phosphine or arsine. So it is necessary to understand the atomic dynamics and interactions which play key role in diverse areas affirmed above.

McEachran and Stauffer [9] have used the relativistic distorted-wave method with multiconfiguration Dirac-Fock wave functions for atomic states of Argon. The distortion potentials with and without a polarization potential were used. The results obtained for distortion potentials without polarization gave good agreement with the experimental measurements for positron impact energies between 20 and 30 eV. An ab initio relativistic calculation has been performed by Sienkiewicz *et al* [10] to search for critical minima in the angle and energy differential cross sections for the elastic scattering of electrons from Argon atoms. The theoretical approach is based on the Dirac–Hartree–Fock method. The exchange between incident and target electrons is calculated exactly. The target polarization is described by an ab initio potential taken from relativistic polarized orbital calculations and comparison is made with experimental data and other theoretical results. Finally, they conclude that their fully relativistic, which incorporates target polarization and exchange effects, gives proper description of minima positions in differential cross section for elastic scattering of electrons from Argon. In order to provide more accurate excitation data Griffin *et al* [11] have completed a 452-term *R*-matrix with pseudo-states (RMPS) calculation of electron-impact excitation for Argon. Using these improved data, they have repeated the modeling studies presented in the earlier papers. They compared their excitation data, as well as the results of the collisional radiative calculations, with those arising from the 40-term R-matrix calculation and found significant differences. Taking into account the completeness property of atomic and molecular wave functions, Kretinin *et al* [12] have proposed a new approximation inelastic electron atom and electron molecule scattering. Thus involving only the ground-state wave function within the framework of the first Born approximation they showed that the calculation of the inelastic total integral cross sections (TICS) for electron scattering by Argon shows asymptotic coincidence with experimental data. Ballance and Griffin [13] have presented the results of the first R-matrix with pseudo states (RMPS) calculation of excitation in neutral Argon. The differential and total excitation cross sections resulting from this RMPS calculation are compared to those from a standard R-matrix calculation without pseudo state. These comparisons indicate that the effects of continuum coupling are large even for transitions from the ground term to the lowest excited terms, although they are most pronounced above the ionization limit, they are still important at lower energies. This demonstrates the need for a full intermediate coupling RMPS calculation between individual levels in Argon, and this will present a formidable computational challenge. McEachran and Stauffer [14] have presented differential scattering cross section with the help of a complex ab initio optical potential calculation for elastic electron and positron scattering from Argon atoms. They showed that inclusion of the absorption part of this potential markedly improves the agreement of their results with experimental measurements for electron and positron different, in various energy ranges. Gangwar *et al* [15] have used the relativistic distorted-wave approximation to calculate the excitation of Argon from its ground state to the higher lying fine-structure levels of the $3p^5 3d$, $3p^5 5s$, and $3p^5 5p$ manifolds. The calculation has been performed with relativistic Dirac-Fock multiconfiguration wave functions for the ground and excited states. Liang *et al* [16] have calibrated the distorted wave Born approximation (DWBA) for electron impact excitation processes empirically and calculated results are compared with the absolute experimental measurements and other theoretical results. Overestimating the magnitude they found that the structure of the DCS can be well reproduced by the DWBA model. Jones *et al* [17] have presented high-resolution measurements of positron interactions with neon and Argon over a range of 0.3 to 60 eV. Comparison among the theoretical treatments of scattering from Neon and Argon by relativistic optical potential approach and calculations using the convergent close coupling method are made also with previous theoretical and experimental work.

Mielewska *et al* [18] have measured differential cross sections for elastic electron scattering in Argon in the angular range of backward scattering from 130° to 180° at low incident electron energies with the help of magnetic angle changing technique with a newly developed conical solenoid. They have also presented a detailed comparison in between differential and integral cross sections obtained with the results of various theoretical calculations. Using a conventional high resolution electron spectrometer, Khakoo *et al* [19] have reported electron impact differential cross-section (DCS) and DCS ratio for the excitation of the four levels making up the $3p^5 4s$ configuration of Argon at incident electron energies of 14, 15, 17.5, 20, 30, 50 and 100 eV. They have used elastic electron scattering from Argon as a calibration standard and electron Helium DCS to determine the instrumental transmission of the spectrometer. Lastly they also presented results from new calculations of these DCS using the *R*-matrix method, the semi-relativistic distorted-wave Born approximation, and relativistic distorted-wave method. Allan *et al* [20] have reported absolute angle-differential cross sections as a function of electron energy up to a few eV above threshold at a fixed scattering angle of 135° for electron-impact excitation of Argon atom to the lowest four $np^5(n+1)s$ levels. They have also compared their results with predictions from a Breit-Pauli *B*-spline *R*-matrix methods, in which nonorthogonal orbital sets are used to optimize the target description. Mondal *et al* [21] have measured electron impact differential cross section of Argon. The scattered electrons are captured over a broad range of energies with constant transmission, thereby eliminating potential source of error in relating relative intensities. Experimental data is compared with new relativistic distorted wave (RDW) calculation. Cho and park [22] have measured the differential cross sections for elastic electron scattering from Argon at backward scattering angles at five incident electron energies from 5 to 50 eV. A magnetic angle-changing device has been used to extend the present measurements from mid-angles to backward angles up to 180^0. A comparison with previous experimental and theoretical results for Argon and with results for other rare gases is presented too. Mondal *et al* [23] have presented absolute differential cross section (DCS) data for the excitation of the $3p^54s$ manifold in Argon by electron impact with the help of experiment based time of flight technique (TOF). Their study focuses on the near threshold region where previous studies have revealed persistent disparities between measurements and theoretical predictions. Through the applications of improved experimental techniques they tried to minimize the gap between experiment and theory. Recently Zecca *et al* [24] have reported results from new positron Argon total cross-section (TCS) measurements. They found agreement with the corresponding recent data of Jones *et al* [17] except at the lowest energies of common measurements. Excellent qualitative agreement is also found between their measurements and an improved convergent close-coupling (CCC) calculation.

The present study concerns the elastic and inelastic scattering of Argon atoms by electron as well as positron, for which discrepancies between experiment and theory have persisted over a number of decades. It is used in a variety of applications including Argon lasers, plasma processing, incandescent lighting, and welding.

4.2   THEORY

4.2.1   ELASTIC SCATTERING

Consider a projectile of charge e_p, with energy E, being scattered elastically by a target with central potential $V(r)$. The scattering can be described by the radial part, $u_l(r)$, of the lth partial wave function which satisfies (in atomic unit)

$$\left[\frac{d^2}{dr^2} - \frac{l(l+1)}{r^2} + 2\mu[E - V(r)]\right]\mu_l(r) = 0 \qquad \text{.... (4.1)}$$

Here μ is the reduced mass of the system. The radial part of asymptotic wave function is

$$\mu_l(r) \underset{r \to \infty}{\longrightarrow} kr[j_l(kr) - (\tan \delta_l)n_l(kr)], \qquad \text{.... (4.2)}$$

where $k^2 = 2\mu E$. j_l and n_l are the spherical Bessel functions of first and second kind, respectively. For positron and electron impact, $\mu = 1$. δ_l is the energy dependent phase shift caused by the potential $V(r)$. From the values of the wave function at two adjacent points r and $r + h$ $(h \ll r)$, in the asymptotic domain, one can extract the phase shift

$$\tan \delta_l = -\frac{(r+h)\mu_l(r)j_l(k(r+h))-r\mu_l(r+h)j_l(kr)}{r\mu_l(r+h)n_l(kr)-(r+h)u_l(r)n_l(k(r+h))} \qquad \text{.... (4.3)}$$

Various phase shifts are used to obtain scattering amplitude as

$$f(\theta) = \frac{1}{2ik}\sum_{l=0}^{\infty}(2l + 1)\left(e^{2i\delta_l} - 1\right)P_l(\cos \theta) \qquad \text{.... (4.4)}$$

where θ is scattering angle. Equation (4.1) is solved by using Numerov procedure and the first L phase shifts are obtained exactly. L depends on the energy of the incident projectile. For large $l(> L)$ the exact phase shifts δ_l are approximately equal to the Born phase shifts δ_{Bl},

$$\exp(i\delta_{Bl})\sin \delta_{Bl} \equiv T_{Bl} = -2k \int_0^{\infty} r^2 j_l^2(kr)V(r)\, dr \qquad \text{.... (4.5)}$$

The infinite sum in equation (4.4) is approximated by

$$f(\theta) = \frac{1}{2ik}\sum_{l=0}^{L}(2l + 1)[exp(2i\delta_l) - 1 - exp(2i\delta_{Bl}) + 1] \times P_l(\cos \theta) + f_B(\theta)$$

$$\text{.... (4.6)}$$

where f_B is the scattering amplitude in the Born approximation. For a spherically symmetric potential $V(r)$,

$$f_B(\theta) = \frac{1}{2ik}\sum_{l=0}^{\infty}(2l+1)\left(e^{2i\delta_{Bl}}-1\right)P_l(\cos\theta) = -2\int_0^{\infty} r^2 \frac{\sin(qr)}{qr} V(r)\,dr$$

$$\text{.... (4.7)}$$

where $q = 2k\sin\frac{\theta}{2}$ is the momentum transfer. The differential and integral elastic cross sections are

$$\frac{d\sigma}{d\Omega} = |f(\theta)|^2, \qquad\qquad\qquad\qquad\qquad\qquad \text{.... (4.8)}$$

$$\sigma_I = 2\pi\int_0^{\infty}\left[\frac{d\sigma}{d\Omega}\right]\sin\theta\,d\theta \qquad\qquad\qquad\qquad \text{.... (4.9)}$$

In the present calculation of elastic scattering of electrons and positrons by Argon atoms, the potentials used are

$$V(r) = V_S(r) + V_P(r) \qquad\qquad \text{for positron impact} \qquad\qquad \text{.... (4.10)}$$

$$V(r) = V_S(r) + V_P(r) + V_{ex}(r) \qquad \text{for electron impact} \qquad\qquad \text{.... (4.11)}$$

Here $V_S(r)$ is the static potential for of the target atom, obtained by averaging over the motion of the target electrons and for Argon it is given by

$$V_S(r) = e_p \sum_{\lambda=1}^{N}\sum_{p=0}^{\lambda-1} N_{\lambda_p}\sum_{i=1}^{M}\sum_{j=1}^{M} a\exp(-zr)\left[\frac{s}{r}+\sum_{t=0}^{\nu-2} mr^t\right] \qquad \text{.... (4.12)}$$

where N is the number of occupied shells in the atom and N_{λ_p} is the number of electrons in the orbital (λ, p). V_p is taken to be a model polarization potential of the Buckingham type

$$V_p(r) = -\frac{1}{2}\alpha\, r^2/(r^2+d^2)^3 \qquad\qquad\qquad\qquad \text{.... (4.13)}$$

where α is the static dipole polarizability. d is an energy dependent adjustable parameter determined by fitting the calculated differential and integral cross section for the elastic scattering of electrons by Argon atoms with the experimental values of the same at a particular energy. The same value of d is then used for positron Argon scattering calculations at that energy. The value of the parameter of d for various impact energies are given by Khare *et al* [25-27] who have used a very similar polarization potential, have expressed the parameter d as a linear function of k in their work. The exchange potential, $V_{ex}(r)$ for a closed shell atom is then taken to be [28-30].

$$V_{ex}(r) = \frac{1}{2}\left[[E - V_D(r)] - \left[[E - V_D(r)]^2 + \sum_{\lambda=1}^{N}\sum_{p=0}^{\lambda-1} N_{\lambda_p}\left|\phi_{\lambda_p}(r)\right|^2\right]^{1/2}\right]$$

.... (4.14)

where V_D is the direct interaction potential, namely $V_D = V_S + V_P$. $\phi_{\lambda_p}(r)$ is the radial part of Slater-type orbital. $V_{ex}(r)$ is a shorter range and much weaker potential than the static potential, hence excluded from the computation of the phase shifts of higher partial waves using the Born approximation.

4.2.2   INELASTIC SCATTERING

In the first Born approximation, when electron with initial momentum P, scatters on the many electron target (atom or molecule), the transition probability from the initial state $|i\rangle$ with energy E_i to the final state $|f\rangle$ with energy E_f is determined by

$$dw_{i\rightarrow f} = 2\pi|\langle f\boldsymbol{P}'|U|i\boldsymbol{P}\rangle|^2\delta\left(\frac{P'^2-P^2}{2} + E_f - E_i\right)\frac{d\boldsymbol{p}'}{(2\pi)^3}$$

.... (4.15)

where $\quad U = \sum_{j=1}^{A}\frac{Z_i}{|r-R_j|} - \sum_{j=1}^{N}\frac{1}{|r-r_j|}$

.... (4.16)

is the interaction potential of the incident electron and the atom composed of a nuclei with charges Z_j, coordinates $\boldsymbol{R}_j$ and N electrons.

The differential cross section (DCS) of electron scattering for the transition from molecular state $|i\rangle$ to state $|f\rangle$ is

$$\frac{d\sigma_{i\rightarrow f}}{d\Omega} = \frac{P'}{4\pi^2 p}\left|\int\langle f|U\,e^{-iqr}|i\rangle d\boldsymbol{r}\right|^2$$

.... (4.17)

where $\boldsymbol{q} = \boldsymbol{p} - \boldsymbol{p}'$ is the electron momentum transfer.

To calculate inelastic DCS one must sum the transitional DCS (4.17) over all final states $|f\rangle$:

$$\frac{d\sigma_r}{d\Omega} = \sum_{f \neq i} \frac{d\sigma_{i \to f}}{d\Omega} \qquad \qquad \text{.... (4.18)}$$

In the adiabatic approach the atomic wave functions depend parametrically on internuclear distance, $\mathbf{R}$, so from the orthogonality of the initial and final states, $\langle f|i\rangle = 0$, it follows that the electron-nucleus interaction turns into zero:

$$\langle f | \frac{Z}{\left|r-\frac{\mathbf{R}}{2}\right|} + \frac{Z}{\left|r+\frac{\mathbf{R}}{2}\right|} |i\rangle = 0 \qquad \qquad \text{.... (4.19)}$$

Let us introduce the mean excitation energy of the inelastic electron scattering, I, which determines the mean momentum of scattered electrons, $\bar{p}' = \sqrt{p^2 - I}$, and the mean momentum transfer, $\bar{q} = \bar{p}' - \bar{p}$. Now in summation over all allowed transitions $|i\rangle \to |f\rangle$ in equation (4.18) one can replace p' and q, which are specific for the concrete transition, by their mean values and remove them from the sum (4.18),

$$\frac{d\sigma_r}{d\Omega} = \frac{4\bar{p}'}{\bar{q}^4} \sum_{f \neq i} \left| \langle f | \sum_{j=1}^{N} e^{-iqr_j} |i\rangle \right|^2 \qquad \qquad \text{.... (4.20)}$$

To calculate equation (4.20), we use the completeness property of the atomic wave functions, $\sum_f |f\rangle\langle f| = \hat{I}$, where $\hat{I}$ is the unit operator,

$$\sum_{f \neq i} \left| \langle f | \sum_{j=1}^{N} e^{-iqr_j} |i\rangle \right|^2 = \sum_{f \neq i} \sum_{j,k=1}^{N} \langle i | e^{iqr_j} |f\rangle\langle f| e^{-iqr_k} |i\rangle$$

$$\simeq \sum_{j,k=1}^{N} \left[\langle i | e^{i\bar{q}(r_j - r_k)} |i\rangle - \langle i | e^{i\bar{q}r_j} |i\rangle\langle i| e^{-i\bar{q}r_k} |i\rangle \right]$$

$$\text{....(4.21)}$$

Since in the Hartree approach the many electron wave function of atom, $|i\rangle = \prod_{j=1}^{N} \phi_j(\mathbf{r_j})$, is expressed through one electron wavefunctions, $\phi_j(\mathbf{r_j})$, all terms in double sum over j and k in equation (4.21) with $j \neq k$ are cancelled, so one easily obtains

$$\sum_{f \neq i} \left| \langle f | \sum_{j=1}^{N} e^{-i\boldsymbol{q}r_j} | i \rangle \right|^2 N[1 - G(\overline{\boldsymbol{q}})], \qquad\qquad \text{.... (4.22)}$$

where

$$G(\overline{\boldsymbol{q}}) = \frac{1}{N} \sum_{j=1}^{N} \left| \langle \phi_j | e^{-i\boldsymbol{q}r_j} | \phi_j \rangle \right|^2 \qquad\qquad \text{.... (4.23)}$$

And the inelastic DCS is the following

$$\frac{d\sigma_r}{d\Omega} = \frac{4N\overline{p}'}{\overline{q}^4 p} [1 - G(\overline{\boldsymbol{q}})] \qquad\qquad \text{.... (4.24)}$$

If for each given $\overline{\boldsymbol{q}}$ the only one electron shell contributes to $G(\overline{\boldsymbol{q}})$ then all one electron matrix elements in the sum in equation (4.23) are considered to be equal and

$$G(\overline{\boldsymbol{q}}) \approx |F(\overline{\boldsymbol{q}})|^2 \qquad\qquad \text{.... (4.25)}$$

The inelastic DCS is averaged over all atomic orientations as

$$\frac{d\tilde{\sigma}_r}{d\Omega} = \frac{1}{2} \int_0^\pi \frac{d\sigma_r}{d\Omega} \sin\theta_q \, d\theta_q \qquad\qquad \text{.... (4.26)}$$

Inelastic total integral cross section is

$$\tilde{\sigma}_r = \frac{4\pi Z}{p^2} \int_0^\pi \sin\theta_{\overline{q}} \, d\theta_{\overline{q}} \int_{(I/p)^2}^{4p^2} [1 - G(\overline{\boldsymbol{q}})] \frac{d\overline{q}^2}{\overline{q}^4} \qquad\qquad \text{.... (4.27)}$$

4.3 RESULT AND DISCUSSION

We have used equation (4.8) to compute the elastic differential scattering cross sections of Argon by impact of electron as well as positron at incident energies 100, 200 and 300 eV respectively. Further the equation (4.26) is used to obtain electron impact inelastic scattering cross sections at incident energies 50 and 100 eV for 4s and 4p states of Argon. The inelastic total integral cross section is also calculated by equation (4.27) at various energies.

4.3.1   ELASTIC SCATTERING

In figures (4.1) to (4.3) we have plotted the present result of differential cross section (DCS) for elastic scattering of Argon by electron impact at incident energies 100, 200 and 300 eV respectively.

The figure (4.1) shows the present results along with the experimental result of Vuskovic and Kurepa [31] as curve L. We have seen from this figure that the present results almost coincide with experimental data. The primary as well as secondary minima held at same position as that in experimental data.

The figure (4.2) depicts the same results as that in figure (4.1) but at 200 eV electron impact energy. Here the available experimental results R of DuBois and Rudd [32] are also plotted. The present results give almost same DCS as experimental data R give.

Figure (4.3) presents the elastic DCS of Argon by 300 eV electron impact energy. For comparison purpose the experimental results J of Bromberg [33] have also been plotted. It is unfortunate that experimental data J is not available for greater than 50^0 scattering angle. But till the data is available the present results are in reasonable agreement with J. Here we may say that a good agreement between present and experimental result encourages that if experiment is done at 300 eV impact energy, the present result shall support the data.

In figures (4.4) to (4.6) we have plotted the present result of differential cross section (DCS) for elastic scattering of Argon by positron impact at incident energies 100, 200 and 300 eV respectively.

The figure (4.4) gives the present result of DCS for elastic scattering of Argon by positron impact at 100 eV. The experimental data G of Hyder *et al* [34] is also plotted. In this figure till 50^0 the experimental data is available without error therefore after 60^0 the error bars are also shown. In this figure we found a good agreement between both results however no other theoretical results is reported till now.

Figures (4.5) and (4.6) present the results of our study of elastic scattering of Argon by positron impact at 200 and 300 eV energy respectively. In both the figures the variation of the DCS is same in both present result as well as experimental result G of Hyder *et al* [34]. If we compare the present result in all three impact energies the magnitude of DCS is decreased. This statement is confirmed by experimental data.

4.3.2　　INELASTIC SCATTERING

In addition to the elastic scattering we have also studied inelastic scattering of Argon by electron impact. The two transitions *viz* 4s and 4p are studied by calculating the DCS as well as total integral cross section (TICS).

4s – Excitation

The figure (4.7) shows our results of 4s excitation of Argon at 50 eV electron energy along with experimental data C of Chutjian and Cartwright [35]. Except in 60^0 to 90^0 scattering angle range the present results are best matched with experimental data. However above 90^0 angles the present results almost coincide with experimental data C showing same position of secondary minima.

Figure (4.8) shows same results of DCS but at 100 eV electron impact energy. It can be seen in this figure that the present results reproduce experimental data till 130^0. Above this angle the present theoretical calculation gives a higher value of cross sections.

4p – Excitation

Figures (4.9) and (4.10) expose our results of 4p excitation of Argon at incident electron energy 50 and 100 eV respectively. For comparison we have plotted the experimental result of Chutjian and Cartwright [35] in both the cases. By observing these two figures we may say that some irregularities are present in our results. However same irregularities can also be seen in experimental data. Therefore more theoretical as well as experimental results are required for this excitation.

Total Integral Cross Section

Figure (4.11) shows the plot of total integral cross sections (TICS) of Argon verses incident electron energy. For comparison we have plotted experimental result Z of Zecca *et al* [36] with the theoretical result I of Inokuti *et al* [37]. Our results are lying in between experimental and theoretical results. The trend is same as that of other curves. It can be seen that as the increase of impact energy the magnitude of TICS decreases rapidaly.

In table – I, we have compared the present calculated integral elastic cross section using equation (4.9) with other available experimental results [38-44]. From this table it can be observed that present calculated values stand within other experimental values very well. It is encouraging feature of present calculation.

4.4   CONCLUDING REMARKS

In conclusion the present calculation provides a reasonable description of physics of the electron and positron elastic scattering by atomic Argon. The total integral cross section (TICS) and differential cross section of Argon by such charged particles are essential sets of data needed in a wide range of applications as discussed in the introduction part of the chapter. More experimental data is needed particularly at higher angle to test the present theoretical understanding properly till the back scattering.

In case of inelastic scattering of Argon by electron, the presence of some irregularity in both the present as well as experimental data, we expect more experimental and sophisticated theoretical data in near future to certify the best sanctity of the present results.

FIGURE CAPTIONS

Figure [4.1]   **: DCS for elastic scattering of Argon by impact of electron at 100 eV**

——————— : Present result

• • • • : Experimental result of Vuskovic and Kurepa [31]

Figure [4.2]   **: DCS for elastic scattering of Argon by impact of electron at 200 eV**

——————— : Present result

• • • • : Experimental result of DuBois and Rudd [32]

Figure [4.3]   **: DCS for elastic scattering of Argon by impact of electron at 300 eV**

——————— : Present result

• • • • : Experimental result of Bromberg [33]

Figure [4.4]   **: DCS for elastic scattering of Argon by impact of positron at 100 eV**

——————— : Present result

• • • • : Experimental result of Hyder *et al* [34]

Figure [4.5]   **: DCS for elastic scattering of Argon by impact of positron at 200 eV**

——————— : Present result

• • • • : Experimental result of Hyder *et al* [34]

DCS FOR ELASTIC SCATTERING OF ARGON BY IMPACT OF ELECTRON AT 100 eV

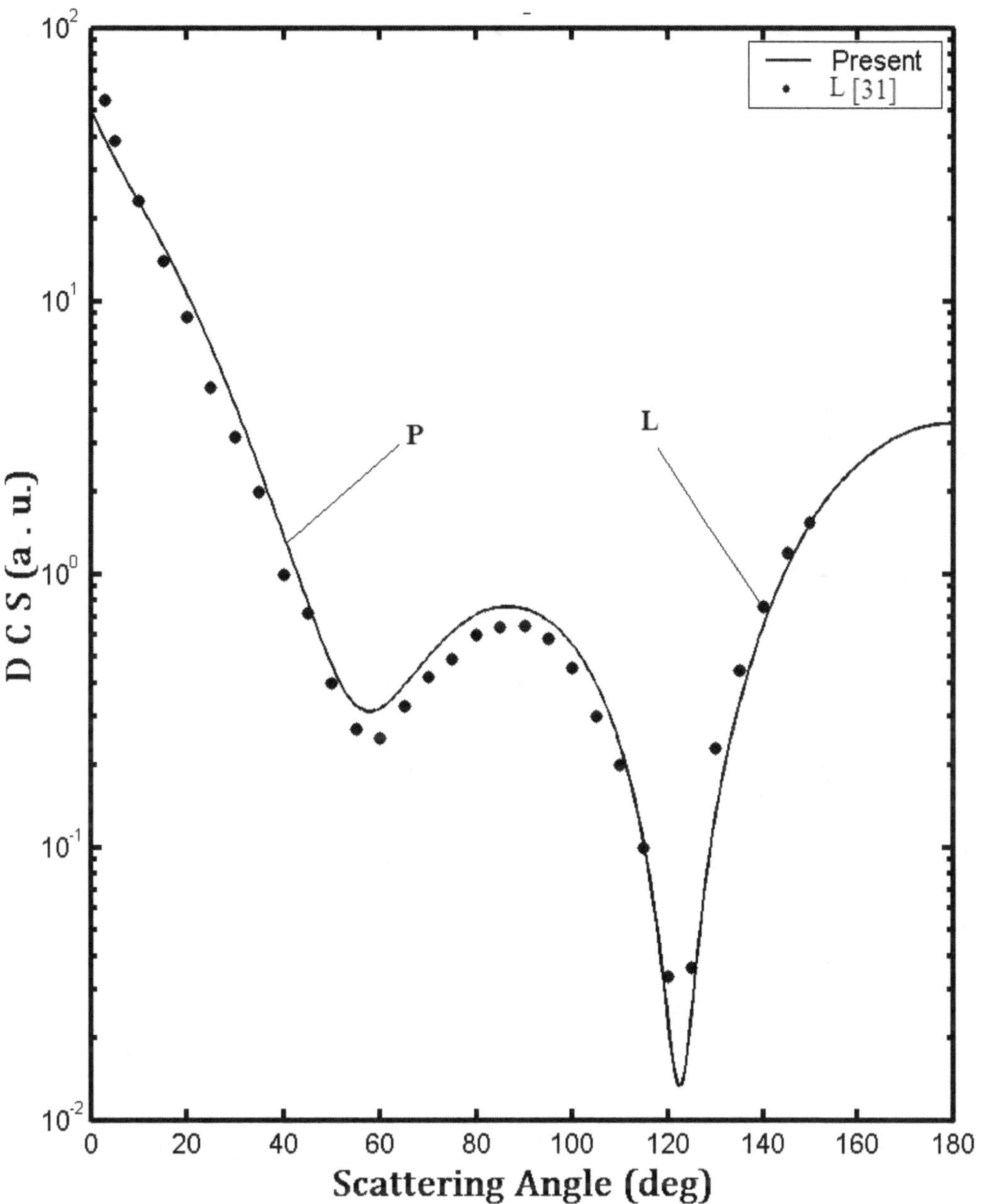

FIGURE [4.1]

DCS FOR ELASTIC SCATTERING OF ARGON BY IMPACT OF ELECTRON AT 200 eV

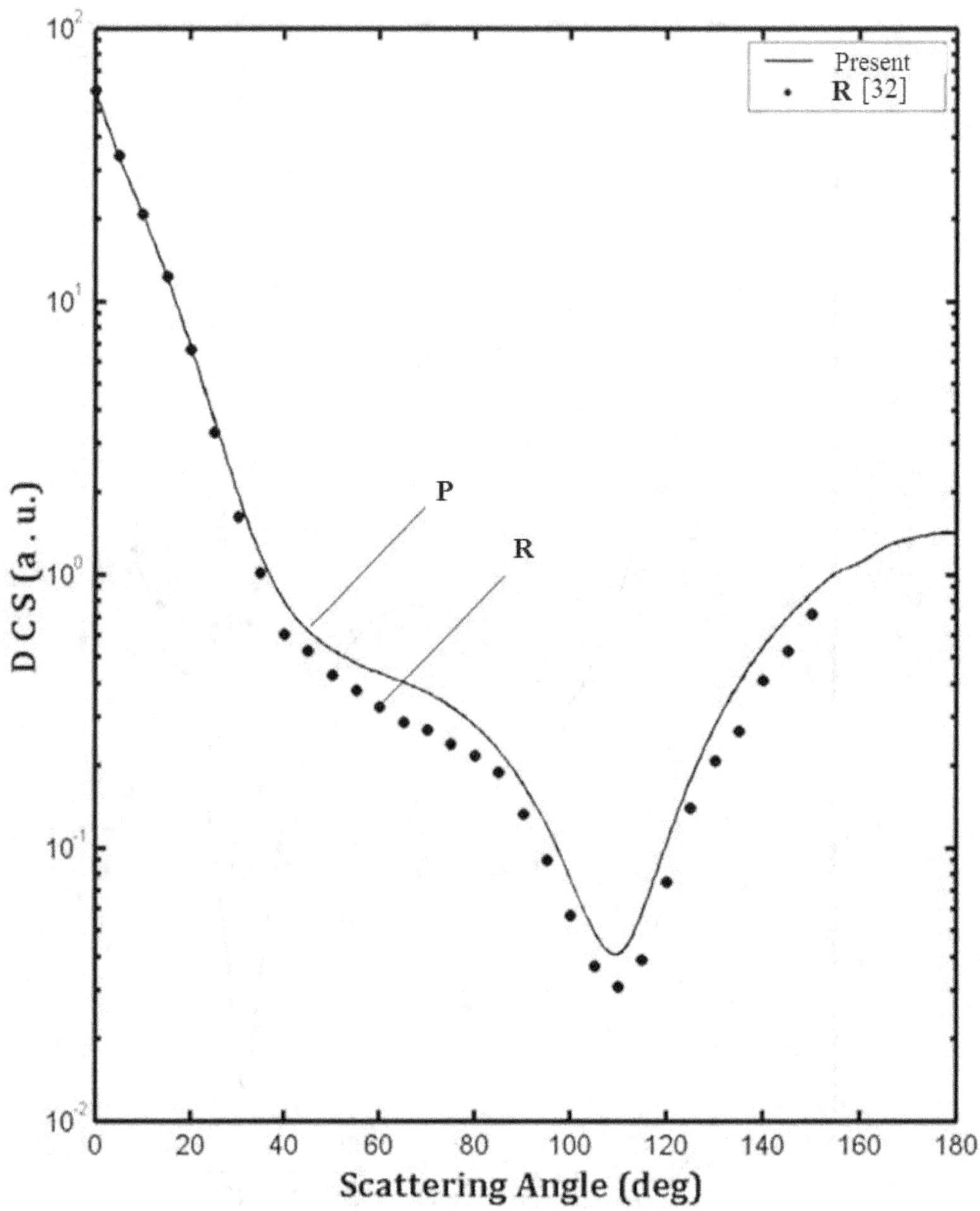

FIGURE [4.2]

DCS FOR ELASTIC SCATTERING OF ARGON BY IMPACT OF ELECTRON AT 300 eV

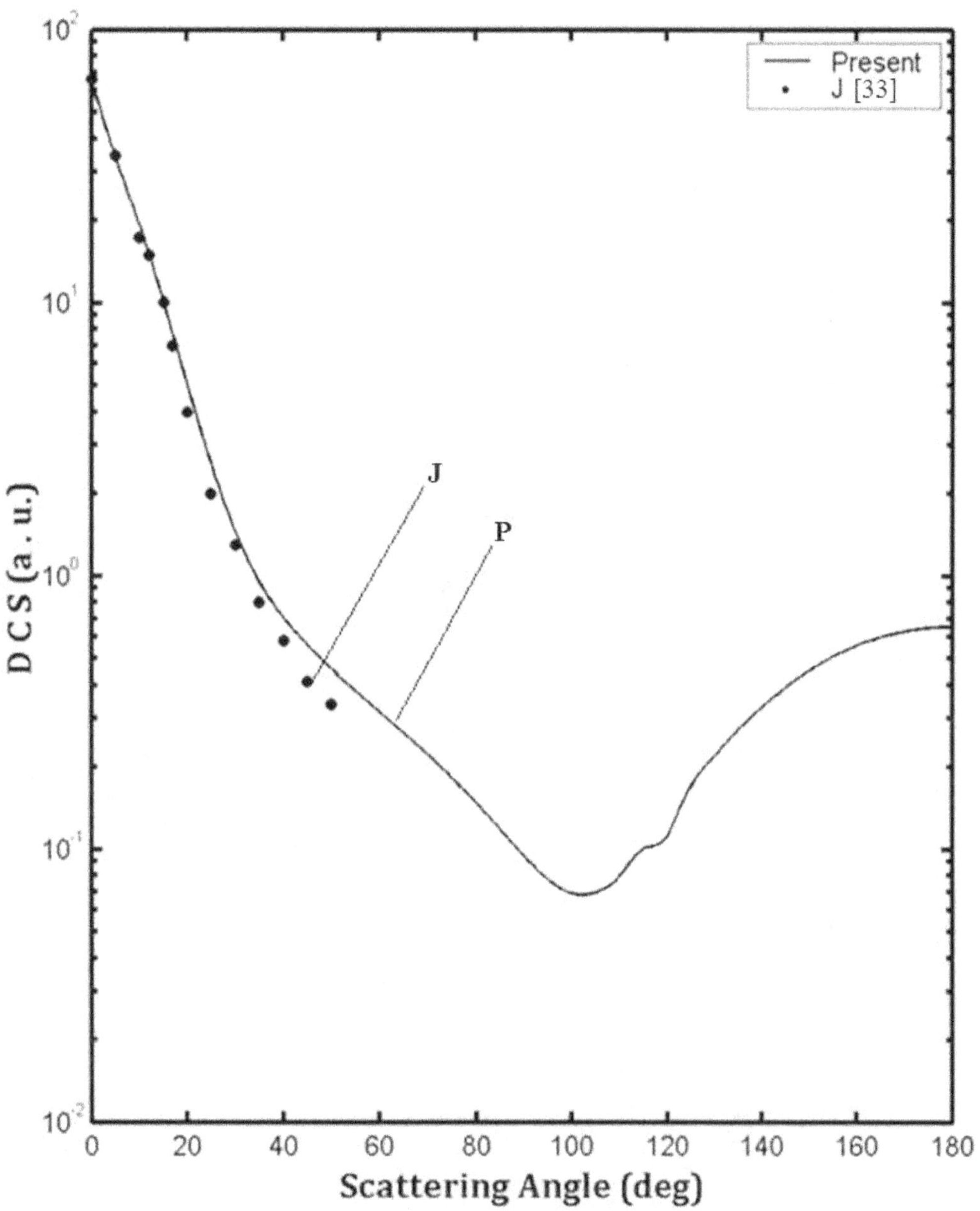

FIGURE [4.3]

DCS FOR ELASTIC SCATTERING OF ARGON BY IMPACT OF POSITRON AT 100 eV

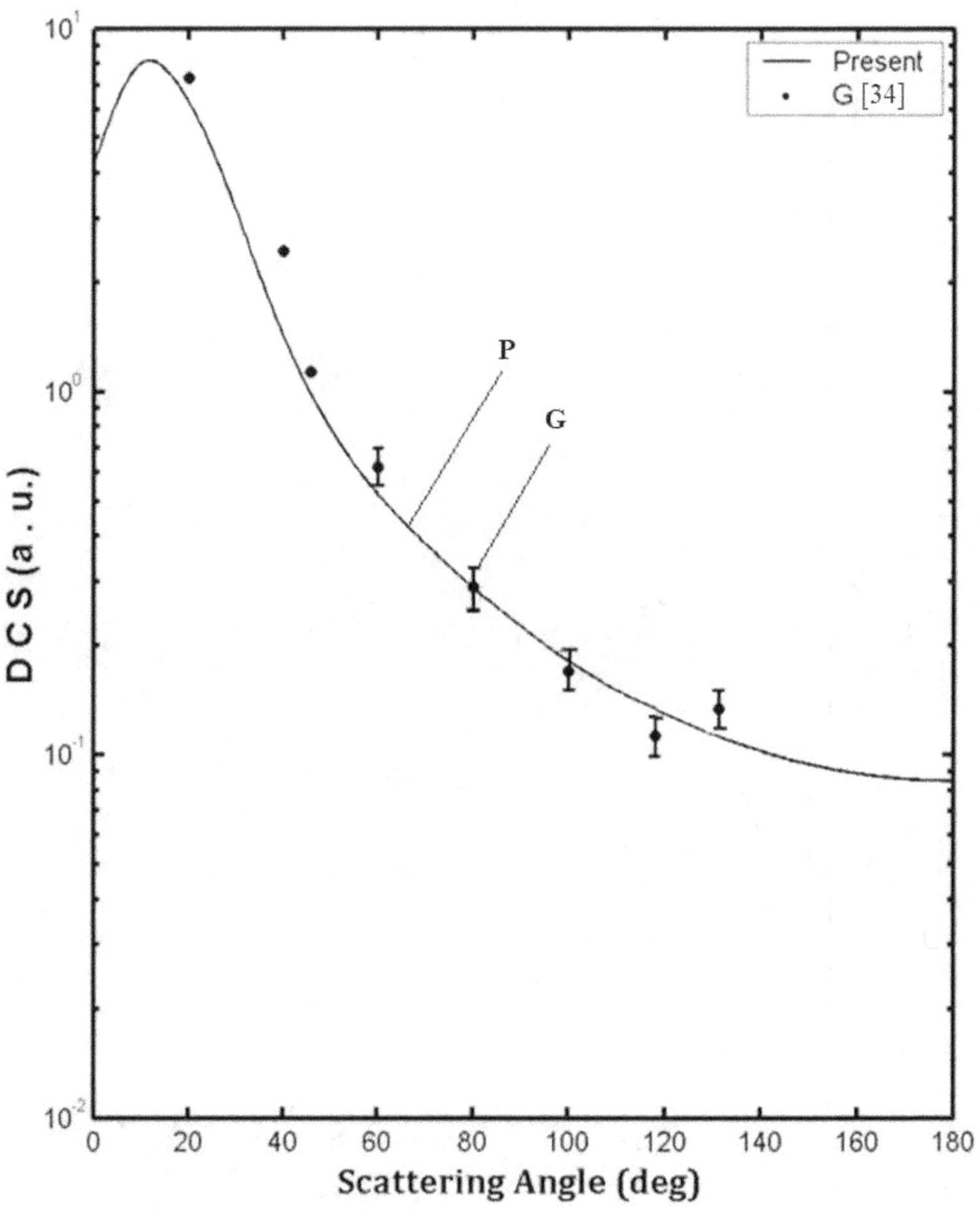

FIGURE [4.4]

DCS FOR ELASTIC SCATTERING OF ARGON BY IMPACT OF POSITRON AT 200 eV

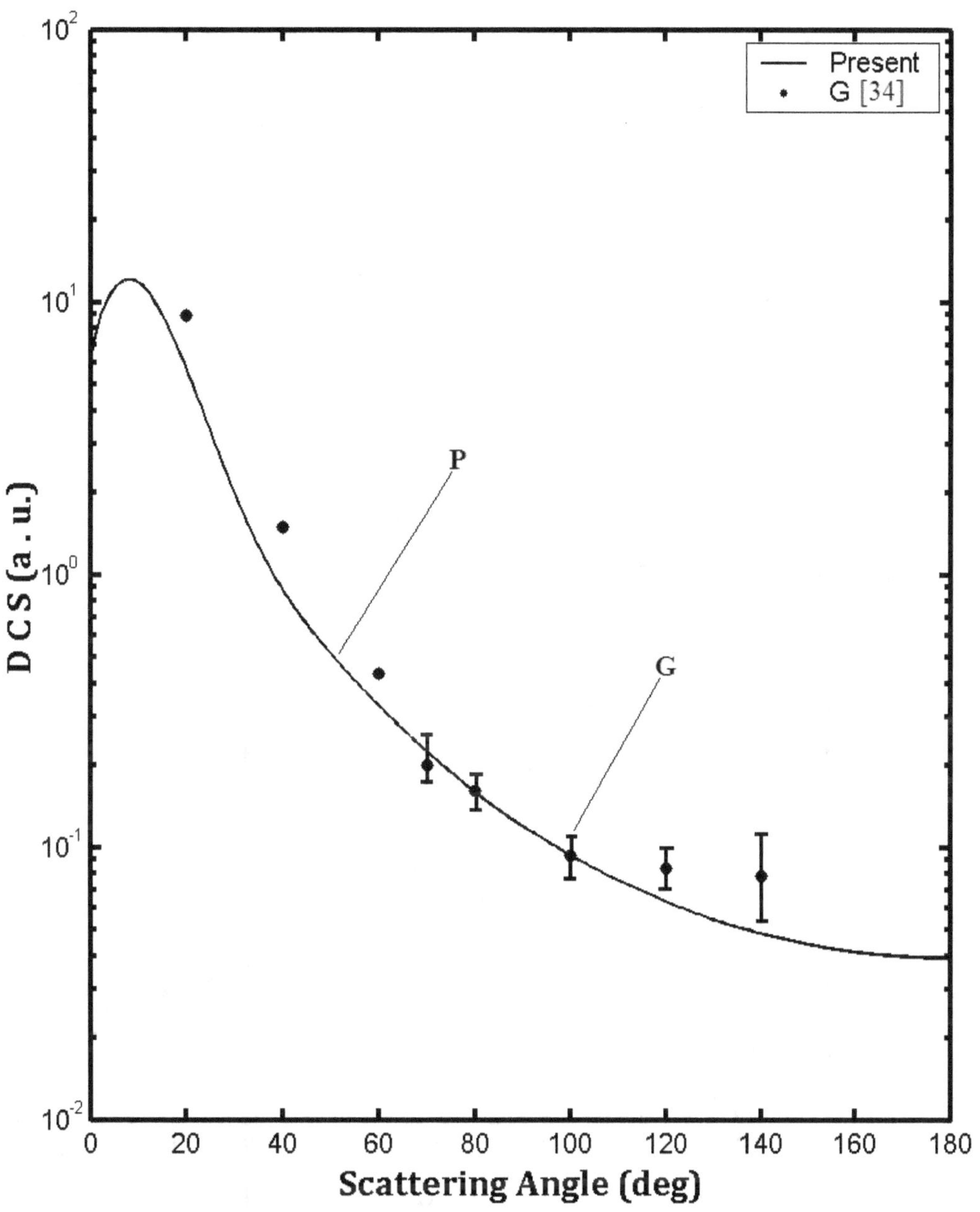

FIGURE [4.5]

DCS FOR ELASTIC SCATTERING OF ARGON BY IMPACT OF POSITRON AT 300 eV

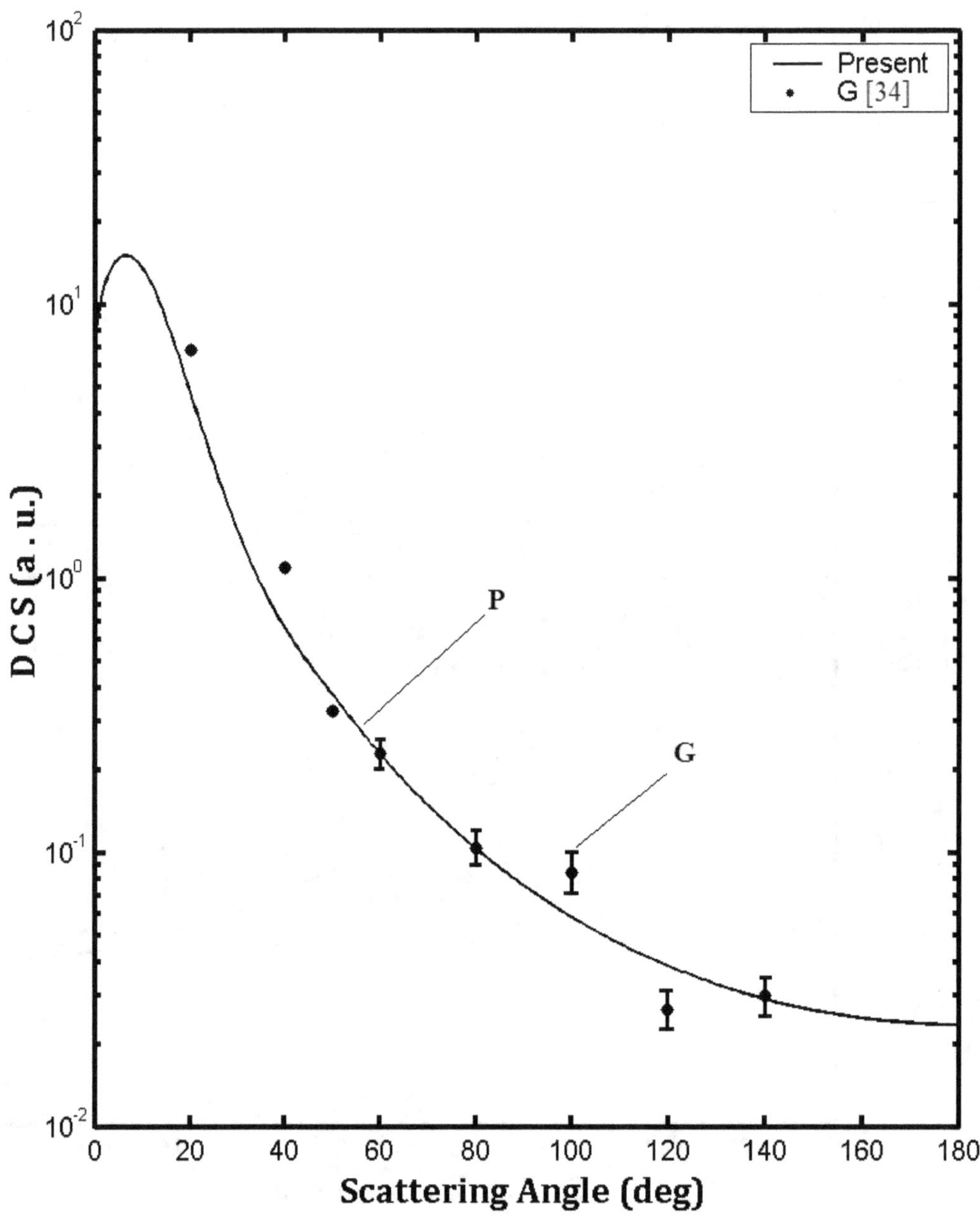

FIGURE [4.6]

DCS FOR (4s) EXCITATION OF ARGON
BY IMPACT OF ELECTRON AT 50 eV

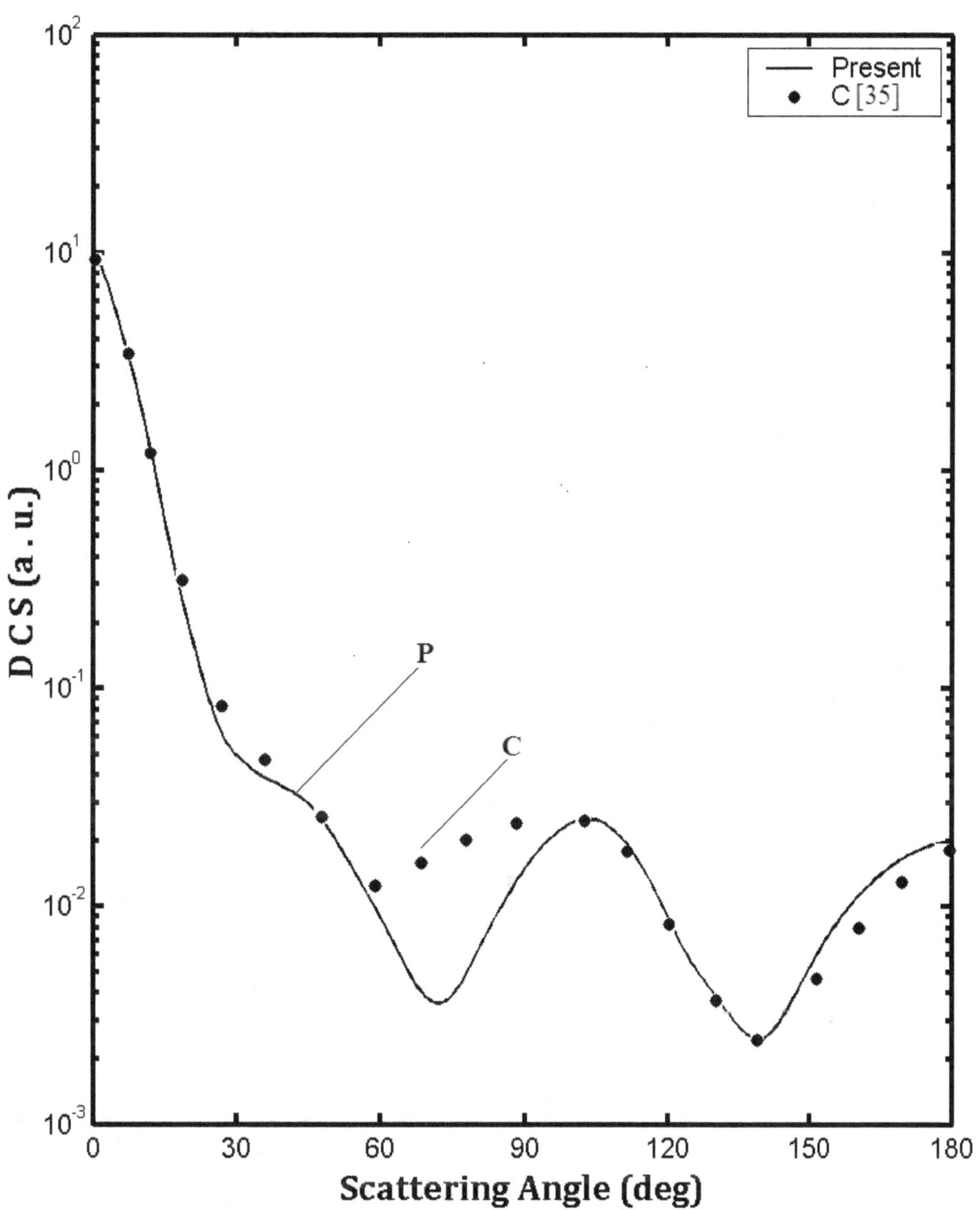

FIGURE [4.7]

DCS FOR (4s) EXCITATION OF ARGON
BY IMPACT OF ELECTRON AT 100 eV

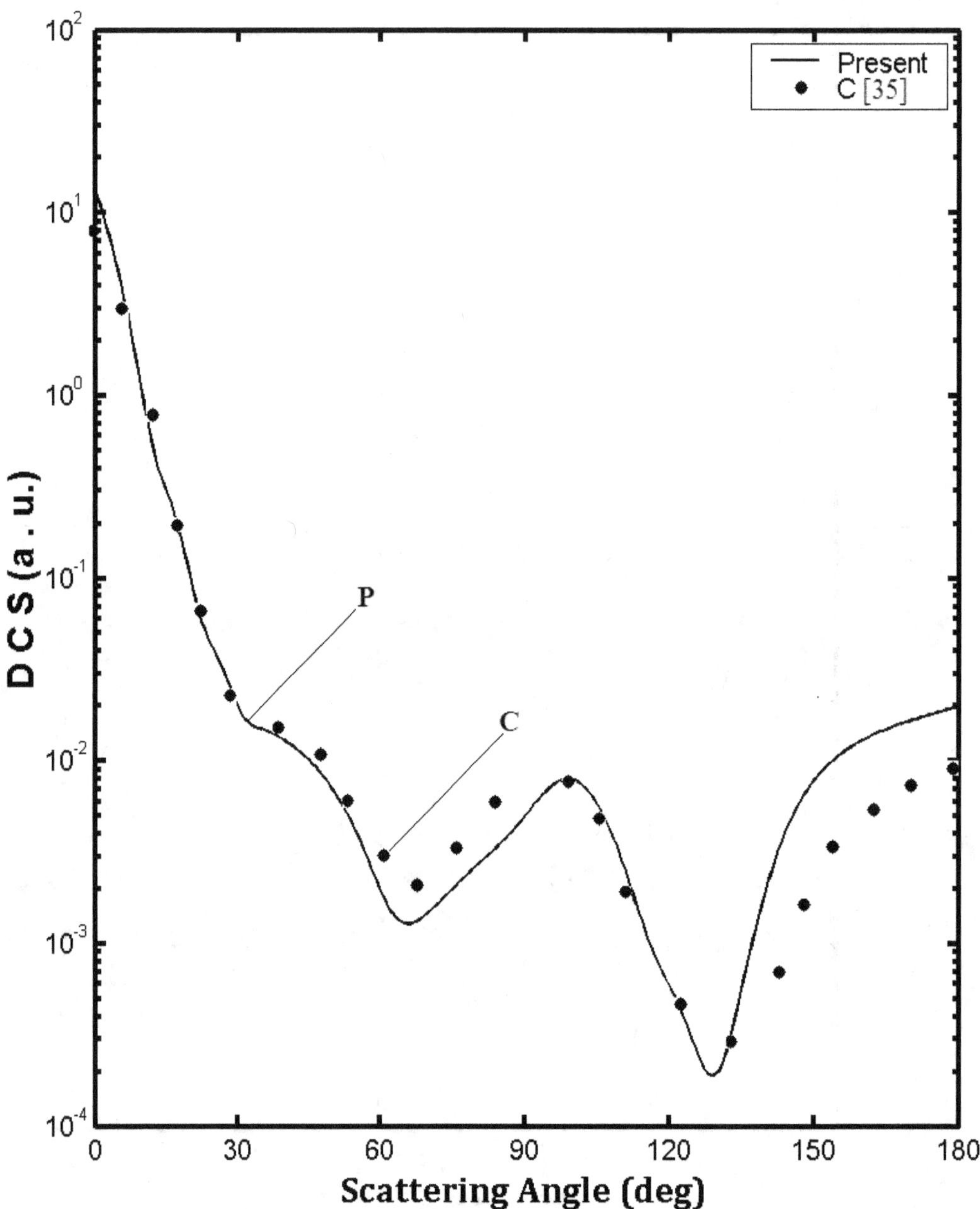

FIGURE [4.8]

DCS FOR (4p) EXCITATION OF ARGON BY IMPACT OF ELECTRON AT 50 eV

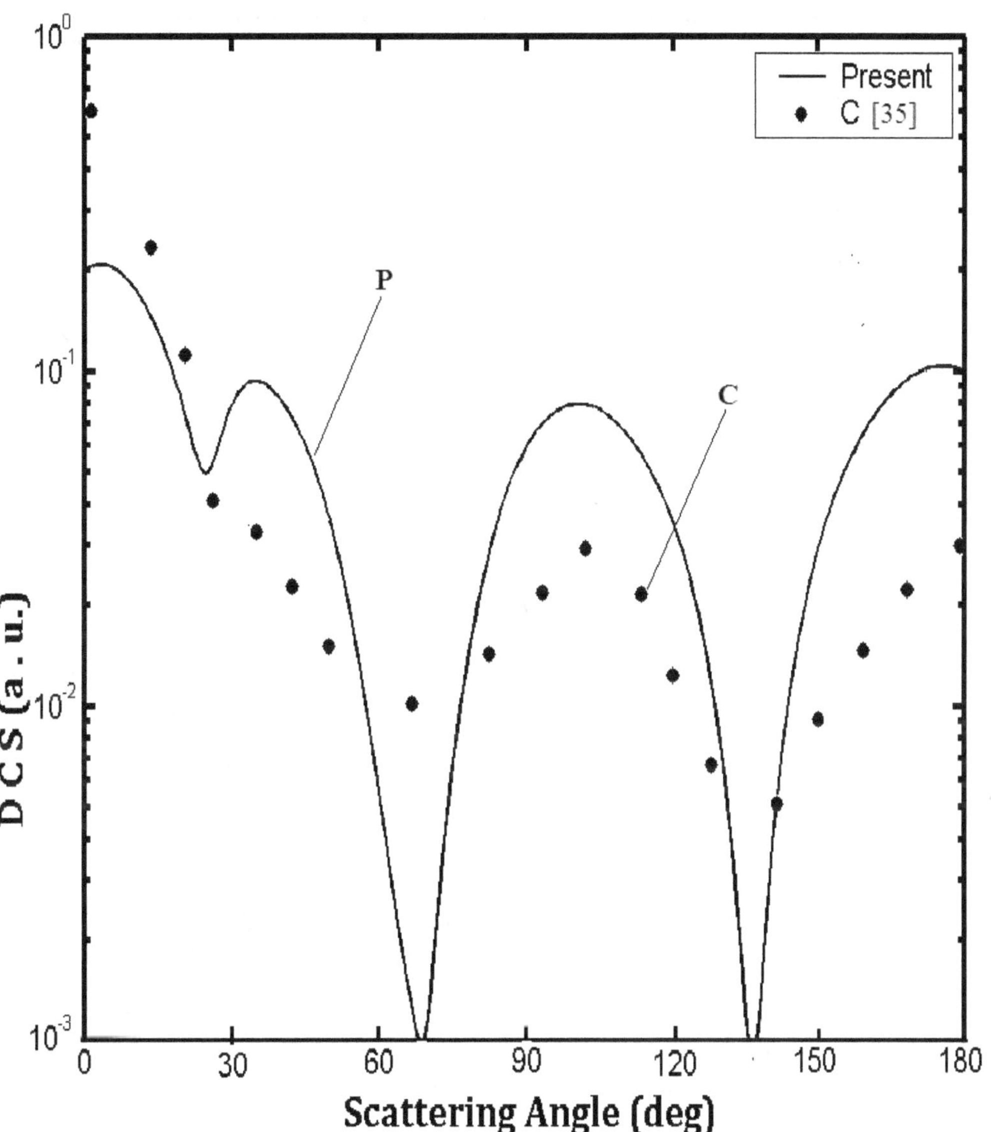

FIGURE [4.9]

DCS FOR (4p) EXCITATION OF ARGON
BY IMPACT OF ELECTRON AT 100 eV

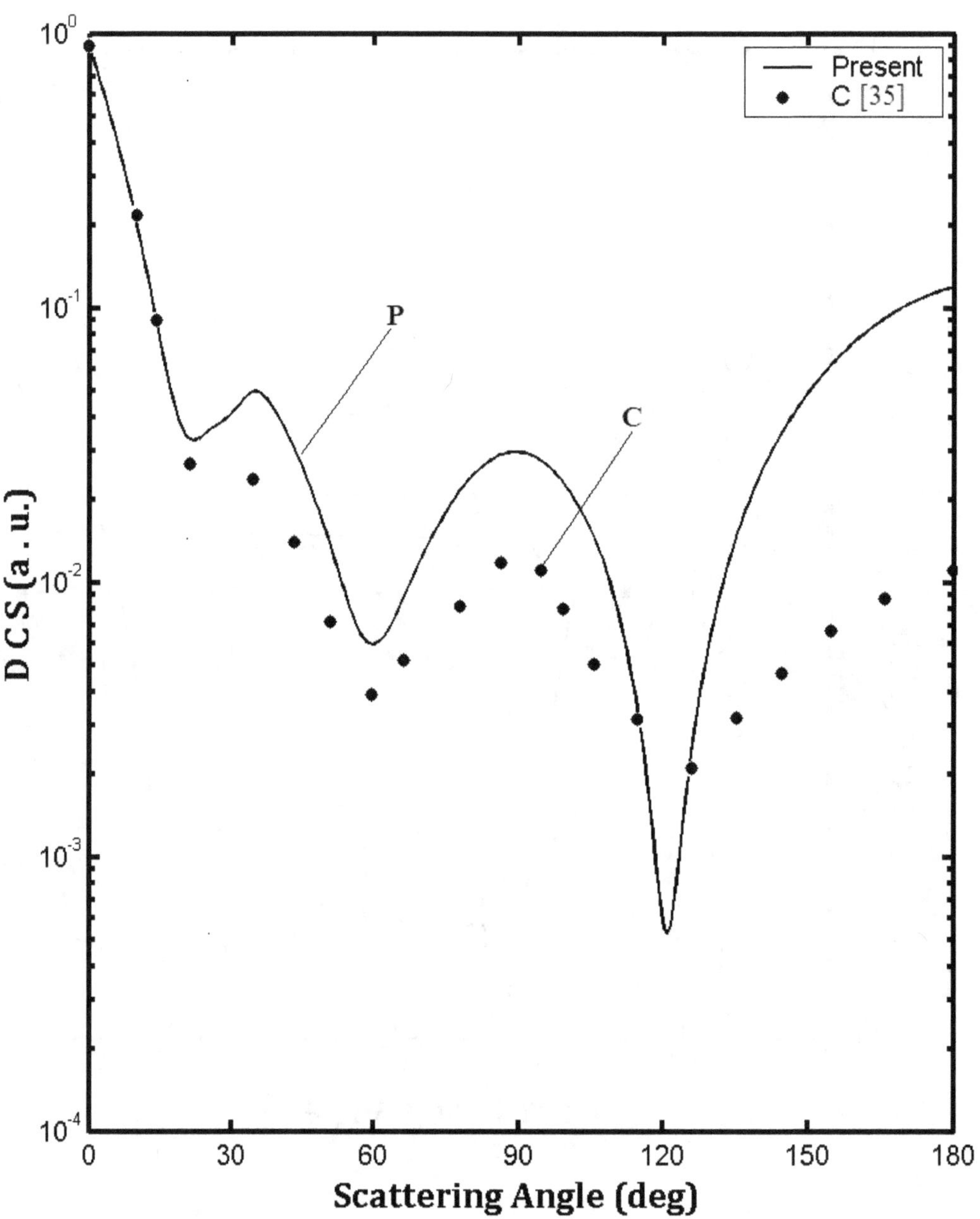

FIGURE [4.10]

TOTAL INTEGRAL CROSS SECTION OF ARGON

BY IMPACT OF ELECTRON

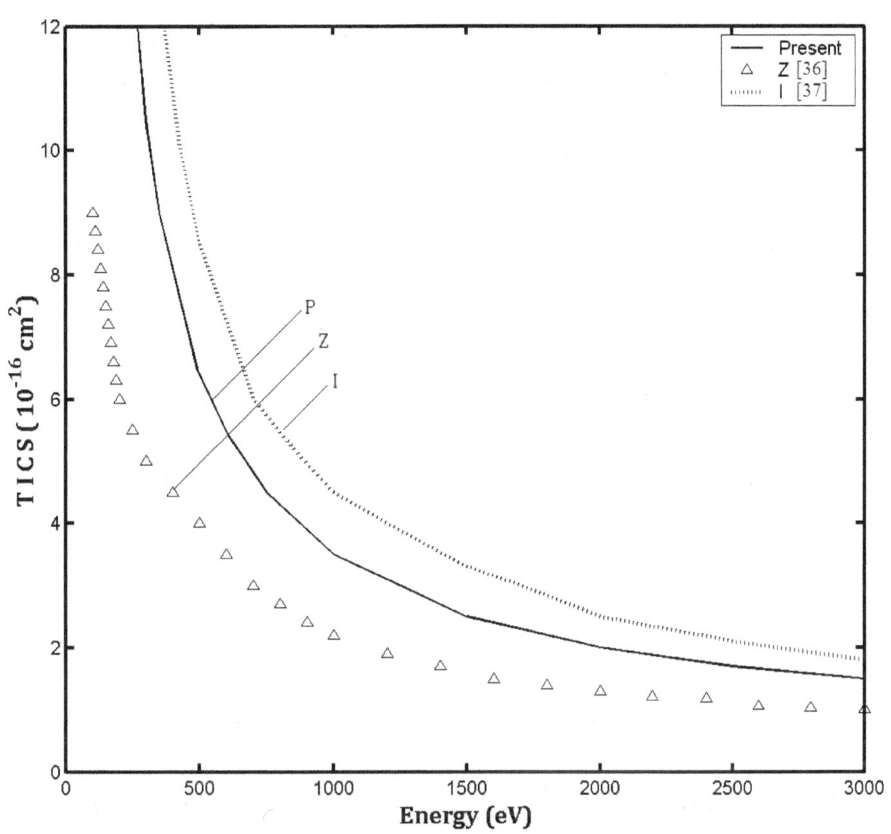

FIGURE [4.11]

TABLE –I

Comparison of calculated integrated elastic cross sections (in units of a_0^2) with experimental values

Projectile	Energy(eV)	Present value	Experimental values
electron	100	19.14	18.66 [38], 16.51[39], 17.33[40], 17.1[41] 18.04[42], 9.29[43]
electron	200	12.7	11.51[44], 9.81[38], 10.9[41], 12.68[42]
electron	300	10.33	8.74[44], 7.82[38], 8.81[39], 10.19[42]

The notation a [b] means measured value of 'a' taken from reference 'b'.

REFERENCES

1. A. S. Ghosh, N. V. Sil and P. Mandal, Phys. Rep **87**, 313 (1982).

2. M. Cherlton, Rep. Prog. Phys **48,** 737 (1985).

3. S. K. Houston and R. J. Drachman, Phys.Rev. A **3**, 47 (1975).

4. J. W. Humberston and R. I. Compeanu, J. Phys. B **13,** 4907 (1980).

5. R. I. Compeanu and J. W. Humberston, J. Phys. B **10**, L153 (1977).

6. A. R.Tancic, M.YaAmusia, N. K. Cherepkov and M. R. Nikolic, Phys. Lett. A **140**, 503 (1989).

7. E. Ficocelli Varracchio, J. Phys. B **23**, L109 (1990).

8. E. Ficocelli Varracchio and V. T. Lamanna, Chem.Phys. Lett. **38,** 101 (1993).

9. R. P. McEachran and A. D. Stauffer, Phys. Rev. A **65**, 034703 (2002) .

10. J. E. Sienkiewicz, S. Telega, P. Syty and S. Fritzsche, Radiation Physics and Chemistry **68**, 285(2003).

11. D .C. Griffin, C. P. Ballance, S. D. Loch and M. S. Pindzola, *J. Phys. B: At. Mol. Opt. Phys.* **40**, 4537 (2007).

12. I. Yu Kretinin, A. V. Krisilov and B. A. Zon ,J. Phys. B: At. Mol. Opt. Phys. **41** , 215206 (2008).

13. C. P. Ballance and D. C. Griffin , *J. Phys. B: At. Mol. Opt. Phys.* **41,** 065201(2008).

14. R. P. McEachran and A. D. Stauffer, J. Phys. B: At. Mol. Opt. Phys. **42**, 075202 (2009).

15.   R. K. Gangwar, L. Sharma, R. Srivastava, and A. D. Stauffer, Phy. Rev. A **81**, 052707 (2010).

16.   Y. Liang, Z. Chen, D. H. Madison and C. D. Lin, J. Phys. B: At. Mol. Opt. Phys. **44**, 085201 (2011).

17.   A.C. L. Jones, C. Makochekanwa, P. Caradonna, D. S. Slaughter, J. R. Machacek, R. P. McEachran, J. P. Sullivan, and S. J. Buckman, Phy.Rev. A **83**, 032701 (2011).

18.   B. Mielewska, I. Linert, G. C. King, and M. Zubek, Phy. Rev. A **69**, 062716 (2004).

19.   M. A. Khakoo, P. Vandeventer, J. G. Childers, I. Kanik, C. J. Fontes, K. Bartschat, V. Zeman, D. H. Madison, S. Saxena, R. Srivastava and A. D. Stauffer, J. Phys. B: At. Mol. Opt. Phys. **37**, 247 (2004).

20.   M. Allan, O. Zatsarinny and K. Bartschat, Phy.Rev. A**74**, 030701(R) (2006).

21.   S. Mondal, J. lower, S. Buckman, R. P. McEachran and G. Garcia, J. of Phy : Conference series **194**, 042027 (2009).

22.   H. Cho and Y. S. Park, Journal of the Korean Physical Society, Vol. **55**, No. **2**, 459 (2009).

23.   S. Mondal, J. Lower, S. J. Buckman, R. P. McEachran1, G. Garcia, O. Zatsarinny and K. Bartschat, PMC Physics B,**2-3** (2009).

24.   A. Zecca, L. Chiari, E. Trainotti, D. V. Fursa, I. Bray, A. Sarkar, S. Chattopadhyay, K. Ratnavelu and M. J. Brunger, J. Phys. B: At. Mol. Opt. Phys. **45**, 015203(2012).

25.   S. P. Khare, A. Kumar, and K. Lata, Indian J. Pure Appl. Phys. **20**, 379 (1982).

26.   S. P. Khare, A. Kumar, and K. Lata, Phys. Rev. A **33**, 2795 (1986).

27.   B. L. Jhanwar and S. P. Khare, Phys. Lett. 50A, 201 (1974).

28.   M. E. Riley and D. G. Truhlar, J. Chem. Phys. **63**, 2182 (1975).

29.   J. B. Furness and I. E. McCarthy, J. Phys. B **6**, 2280 (1973).

30.   B. H. Bransden, M. R. C. McDowell, C. J. Noble, and T. Scott, *ibid.* **9**, 1301 (1976).

31.   L. Vuskovic and M. V. Kurepa, J. Phys. B **9**, 837 (1976).

32.   R. D. DuBois and M. E. Rudd, J. Phys. B **9**, 2657 (1976).

33.   J. P. Bromberg, J. Chem. Phys. **61**, 963 (1974).

34.   G. M. A. Hyder, M. S. Dababneb, Y. F. Hsieh, W. E. Kauppila, C. K. Kwan, M. Mahdavi-Hezaveh, and T. S. Stein, Phys. Rev. Lett. **57**, 2252 (1986).

35.   A. Chutjian and D. C. Cartwright, Phys. Rev. A **23**, 2178(1981).

36.   A. Zecca *et al*, J. Phys. B: At. Mol. Phys. **20**, 5157 (1987).

37.   M. Inokuti, R.P.Saxon and J. L. Dehmer, Int. J. Radiat. Phys. Chem. **7**, 109 (1975).

38.   J. F. Williams and B. A. Willis, J. Phys. B **8**, 1670 (1975).

39.   R. H. J. Jansen, F. J. de Heer, H. J. Luyken, B. van Wingerden, and H. J. Blaauw, J. Phys. B **9**, 185 (1976).

40.   L. Vuskovic and M. V. Kurepa, J. Phys. B **9**, 837 (1976).

41.   R. D. DuBois and M. E. Rudd, J. Phys. B **9**, 2657 (1976).

42.   S. C. Gupta, Ph.D. thesis, University of Liverpool, 1975.

43.   S. K. Srivastava, H. Tanaka, A. Chutjian, and S. Trajmar, Phys. Rev. A **23**, 2156 (1981).

44.   J. P. Bromberg, J. Chern. Phys. **61**, 963 (1974).

CHAPTER-5

ELECTRON IMPACT EXCITATION OF KRYPTON

5.1 INTRODUCTION

Interaction between an electron beam and a volume of gas may lead to elastic and inelastic excitation of the gas atoms. The probability that a given atom will exhibit a specific reaction due to a collision with a specific kind of incident particle and its energy can be formulated using a classical constructed term the 'cross section'. Atomic or molecular cross sections for excitation to bound states can be determined by examining the wavelengths of light emitted after the interaction has occurred. The cross sections as a function of the bombardment energy or scattering angle are termed excitation function and such data for specific situation are useful as a basis for development of lasing predictions for certain gases. They can also be used to determine the utility of a gas as a particular wave length source. The cross sections are also needed for the theoretical analysis of astrophysical phenomena. Electron impact excitation studies of noble gas atoms are an essential aspect of atomic physics because of their contribution to the knowledge of atomic structure and scattering processes. Moreover, electron impact excitation of heavy rare gases continues to attract great interest in collision physics for several reasons. Recent advances in computer technology have enabled large electron scattering codes to be executable, resulting in more accurate models for electron impact excitation of *LS*-coupled target atoms. Accurate atomic data such as electron impact collision cross sections and electron excitation rates are some of the data required for plasma diagnostic, plasma modeling and also in laser research in soft X-ray region. The past few years are witness of dramatic increase in research studies on low energy scattering of electron from atomic and molecular target due to corresponding improvements in the technology for producing reliable electron beams. The inelastic scattering of electrons by atoms and molecules is of widespread importance in many applications because of its requirement as reference values in applications such as radiation dosimetry, radiation therapy, radiation processing, radiation sensors, and radiation protection to electron-beam lithography, plasma physics, and materials analysis by techniques such as electron-probe microanalysis (EPMA), analytical electron microscopy (AEM), auger electron spectroscopy (AES), and X-ray photoelectron spectroscopy (XPS). For these applications, knowledge of inelastic scattering cross sections can be needed to obtain information on the spatial distribution of energy deposition, to enable more accurate analyses, or to define the analytical volume. More specifically, data for differential scattering cross sections, total elastic-scattering cross sections, transport cross sections, or phase shifts may be required. For crystalline solids, coherent scattering by the ordered atoms leads to electron diffraction, a powerful tool for obtaining information on the atomic structure. Atomic inelastic-scattering cross sections can be used for general applicability in the world of atomic and molecular field. There can be noticeable differences among cross-section data from the different method of calculation but comparison by two or more independent experimental sets of data prove the superiority. The past few years have witnessed a dramatic increase in research studies on scattering of electron from atomic and molecular targets. This increased activity is partly due to corresponding improvements on the technology for producing reliable electron beams. Nevertheless there are still considerable uncertainties in agreement between measured values of electron-atom cross sections.

Krypton was discovered by William Ramsay and M.W. Travers in 1898. The element was named Krypton, after the Greek word kryptos which means hidden. Krypton in trace quantities is found in the earth's atmosphere at a concentration level of about 1.14 ppm. The gas also is found in the spent fuel from nuclear reactors, resulting from fission of Uranium and Plutonium nuclei. Krypton has been found in Mars' atmosphere in trace concentration. The commercial applications of Krypton are fewer than those of helium or argon. Its principal use is in fluorescent lights. It is mixed with argon as a filling gas to enhance brightness of fluorescent tubes. Other applications are in flash tubes for high-speed photography and incandescent bulbs. Radioactive Kr-85 is used as a tracer to monitor surface reactions. The unit of length, meter was previously defined in terms of the orange-red spectral line of Kr-86. Most Krypton produced in commercial scale comes from air. Krypton and other inert gases are obtained from air by a distillation-liquefaction process. Krypton also may be recovered from spent fuel rods of nuclear power plants. It is produced, along with Xenon, in fission of Uranium and Plutonium. This process, however, is not a major source of Krypton, and the recovered gas also contains radioactive Kr-85 isotope.

McEachran and Stauffer [1] have presented differential cross sections for elastic scattering of electrons from Krypton by comparing their results with experimental measurements for differential and integrated cross sections including recent experiments which extend the measurements to larger scattering angles. Their calculations are based upon the relativistic polarized-orbital method and include both static and dynamic polarization potentials as well as an absorption potential to simulate the loss of flux into other channels. The inclusion of these absorption effects significantly improves upon their own previous calculations of the differential cross sections as well as the total and momentum transfer cross sections over the energy range from 10 to 200 eV. Total electron scattering cross sections have been reported by Ariyasinghe and Goains [2] for Krypton at 250–4500 eV electrons by measurement of the electron-beam intensity attenuation through a gas cell. These cross sections are compared with the previous experimental measurements and the predictions by theoretical and semi empirical models. The discrepancies in experimental cross sections between different experimental groups are explained using the oscillator strengths and inelastic threshold of electron energy loss spectra. They have discussed correlation between the total electron scattering cross section and the atomic radius. The electron impact excitation cross sections of Krypton at low electron energies have been calculated by Zeng *et al* [3] using a fully relativistic *R*-matrix method for transitions between levels of $4p^6$, $4p^55s$, and $4p^55p$ configurations. To ensure the convergence of results, they have paid special attention to the factors that may affect the convergence of cross sections. For examples, extensive configuration interactions in the wave-function expansion of the target states have been included. A large enough *R*-matrix boundary has been taken to ensure the convergence of atomic wave functions. The contributions to the cross sections from a large number of partial waves (up to *J*=39.5) have been explicitly calculated. The final results are in good agreement with recent experimental data by Jung *et al.* [4] after shifting the position of electron energy. The relative difference is about 10% for four transitions out of the metastable levels. Bartschat and Zatsarinny [5] have used the *B*-spline *R*-matrix method with non orthogonal orbitals to perform new calculations for the spin asymmetry function S_A, which determines the left–right asymmetry in the differential cross section, for electron impact excitation of the $(3p^54s)^{3,1}P_1$ states in Argon and all four $(4p^5\,5s)$ states in Krypton. Using non-relativistic one-electron orbitals, relativistic effects were accounted for perturbatively through terms of the Breit–Pauli Hamiltonian. In contrast to all previous theoretical attempts, they finally obtain good agreement with the benchmark measurements performed by Dummler *et al* [6]. Chen *et al* [7] have derived a non-local, complex and ab initio absorption potential within the framework of the relativistic Dirac scattering equations and applied it to elastic scattering of electrons and positrons from the heavy noble gases. They have also developed a perturbation method based on the Hulthen–Kato formalism that enables calculations of scattering phase shifts using only real quantities and with a very significant reduction in computational effort. They have used this method to calculate differential cross sections and spin asymmetry parameters for the elastic scattering of electrons from Krypton. In addition, they have applied this method to the elastic scattering of positrons from Krypton and results are compared to experimental measurements. Kretinin *et al* [8] have proposed a new approximation in the theory of inelastic electron–atom and electron–molecule scattering. Taking into account the completeness property of atomic and molecular wavefunctions, considered in the Hartree approximation, and using Bethe's parametrization for electronic excitations during inelastic collisions via the mean excitation energy, they showed that the calculation of the inelastic total integral cross-sections (TICS), in the framework of the first Born approximation, involves only the ground-state wavefunction. The final analytical formula obtained for the TICS, *i.e.* for the sum of elastic and inelastic ones, contains no adjusting parameters. The calculated TICS for electron scattering by light atoms and molecules (He, Ne, and H_2) are in good agreement within the experimental data; results show asymptotic coincidence for heavier ones (Ar, Kr, Xe and N_2). Griffin and Balance [9] have reported the first fully relativistic *R*-matrix calculations with radiation damping for the Helium like ions $Fe24^+$ and $Kr34^+$. The effective collision strengths for these ions have been determined with and without damping over a wide temperature range for all transitions between the 49 levels through $n = 5$. They found that damping has a pronounced effect on the effective collision strengths for excitation to some of the low lying levels, but its effect on excitation to the vast majority of levels is small. At the energy of a resonance peak, they also investigate the effect of radiation damping on the angular distribution of scattered electrons. Zatsarinny and Bartschat [10] have used recently developed semi-relativistic Breit–Pauli and fully relativistic Dirac–Coulomb versions of the *B*-spline *R*-matrix (close-coupling) approach with non-orthogonal orbitals to calculate electron-impact excitation of the $4p^5 5s$ states in Krypton. The comparison of the predictions shows a substantial improvement in the agreement between theory and experiment over that achieved in previous semi-relativistic Breit–Pauli *R*-matrix calculations. In a joint experimental and theoretical effort, Hoffmann *et al* [11] have carried out a detailed study of electron scattering from Krypton atoms in the energy range. The absolute angle-differential cross sections for elastic electron scattering were measured over the energy range 9.3–10.3 eV with an energy width of about 13 M eV at scattering angles between 10^0 and 180^0. Using several sets of elastic scattering phase shifts, a detailed analysis of the sharp Krypton ($4p^5 5s^2$ 2P3/2) resonance was carried out, resulting in a resonance width. In order to obtain additional insights, *B*-spline *R*-matrix calculations were performed for both the elastic and the inelastic cross sections above the threshold for $4p^5$ 5s excitation. They provide the total and angle-differential cross sections for excitation of long-lived and short-lived levels of the $4p^5$ 5s configuration in Krypton and branching ratios for the decay of the Krypton ($4p^5$ $5s^2$ 2P1/2) resonance into the three. Using magnetic angle-changing technique, Linert *et al* [12] have been measured differential cross sections for elastic electron scattering in Krypton at the energies of 5, 7.5, and 10 eV over the scattering angle range from 30^0 to 180^0. They have integrated the measured differential cross sections to yield the elastic integral and momentum transfer cross sections at the same energies. They have also shown dependency of the differential cross sections on atomic polarizability of the heavier rare gas atoms Argon, Krypton, and Xenon over the electron energy range 5–30 eV and for forward, backward, and intermediate scattering angles. Allan *et al* [13] have presented results from a detailed study of electron impact excitation of the $4p^5$ 5s states of Krypton. Very satisfactory agreement between their absolute, high-resolution experimental data and predictions from a fully relativistic DBSR69 model was obtained. The experimental angular distributions extending over the entire angular range were used to derive assumption-free integral cross sections. They agree well with the predictions from both theoretical models.

5.2   THEORY

We consider electron scattering by inert gas containing N electrons and with nuclear charge $Z(=N)$. Denoting the position vector of the ith electron relative to the atomic nucleus by $r_p(r_i)$ the Hamiltonian, H, for this system may be written as

$$H = -\frac{1}{4}\nabla^2_{R_0} + H_{PS}(t_0) + H_A(r_1, \dots . r_N) + V(r_p, r_0, r_1, \dots . r_N) \qquad \text{.... (5.1)}$$

H_{PS} is the electron Hamiltonian,

$$H_{PS}(t) = -\nabla_t^2 - \frac{1}{t} \qquad \qquad \text{.... (5.2)}$$

H_A is the atomic Hamiltonian,

$$H_A(r_1, \ldots r_N) = \sum_{i=1}^{N} \left(-\frac{1}{2}\nabla_i^2 - \frac{Z}{r_i} + \sum_{j<i} \frac{1}{|r_i - r_j|} \right) \qquad \qquad \text{.... (5.3)}$$

and V is the interaction between electron and atom,

$$V(r_p, r_0, r_1, \ldots r_N) = \left(\frac{Z}{r_p} - \sum_{i=1}^{N} \frac{1}{|r_p - r_i|} \right) - \left(\frac{Z}{r_0} - \sum_{i=1}^{N} \frac{1}{|r_0 - r_i|} \right) \qquad \text{.... (5.4)}$$

In the frozen target approximation we expand the collisional wavefunction for the system ψ as

$$\psi = \mathcal{A} \sum_a G_a(R_0)\phi_a(t_0)\chi(s_0)\psi_0(x_0, \ldots x_N) \qquad \qquad \text{.... (5.5)}$$

$\mathcal{A}$ is the electron antisymmetrization operator, the sum is over electron states ϕ_a, ψ_0 is the (normalized) ground state of frozen atomic target, $x_i \equiv (r_i, s_i)$ stands for the space (r_i) and spin (s_i) coordinates of the ith electron and $\chi(s_i)$ is the spin function for the ith electron ($=\alpha$ or β in the usual notation). The function G_a specifies the motion of the electron centre of the mass when it is in the state ϕ_a.

It is assumed that the set of states ϕ_a diagonalizes the electron Hamiltonian $i.e.$

$$\left. \begin{aligned} \langle\phi_a(t)|H_{ps}(t)|\phi_{a'}(t)\rangle &= E_a\delta_{aa'} \\ \langle\phi_a(t)|\phi_{a'}(t)\rangle &= \delta_{aa'} \end{aligned} \right\} \qquad \qquad \text{.... (5.6)}$$

For the atomic ground state ψ_0 we use the Hartree-Fock wavefunctions of Clementi and Roetti [14]. Then ψ_0 has the form

$$\psi_0(x_1, \ldots x_N) = \frac{1}{\sqrt{n!}} \begin{vmatrix} \phi_1(x_1) & \cdot & \cdot & \cdot & \phi_1(x_N) \\ \cdot & & & & \cdot \\ \cdot & & & & \cdot \\ \cdot & & & & \cdot \\ \phi_N(x_1) & \cdot & \cdot & \cdot & \phi_1(x_N) \end{vmatrix} \qquad \qquad \text{.... (5.7)}$$

where the $\phi_i(x)$ are orthonarmal one electron spin orbitals.

The antisymmetrization implied in (5.5) is easily carried out explicitly,

$$\psi = \sum_{a'} \left[\sum_a G_{a'}(\boldsymbol{R}_0)\phi_{a'}(\boldsymbol{t}_0)\chi(s_0)\psi_0(\boldsymbol{x}_1, \dots \boldsymbol{x}_N) \right]$$

$$- \sum_{i=1}^{N} \sum_a G_{a'}(\boldsymbol{R}_i)\phi_{a'}(\boldsymbol{t}_i)\chi(s_i)\psi_0(\boldsymbol{x}_1, \dots \boldsymbol{x}_{N-1},\boldsymbol{x}_0,\boldsymbol{x}_{i+1}, \dots \boldsymbol{x}_{N,}) \qquad \dots (5.8)$$

To obtain coupled equations for G_a, we substitute (5.8) in to Schrödinger equation and project with $\phi_a(\boldsymbol{t}_0)\chi(s_0)\psi_0(\boldsymbol{x}_1, \dots \boldsymbol{x}_N)$, this gives

$$\sum_{a'} [\langle\phi_a(\boldsymbol{t}_0)\chi(s_0)\psi_0(\boldsymbol{x}_1, \dots \boldsymbol{x}_N)|H - E| \sum_a G_{a'}(\boldsymbol{R}_0)\phi_{a'}(\boldsymbol{t}_0)\chi(s_0)\psi_0(\boldsymbol{x}_1, \dots \boldsymbol{x}_N)\rangle$$

$$-N\langle\phi_a(\boldsymbol{t}_0)\chi(s_0)\psi_0(\boldsymbol{x}_1, \dots \boldsymbol{x}_N)|H - E| \times \sum_a G_{a'}(\boldsymbol{R}_1)\phi_{a'}(\boldsymbol{t}_1)\chi(s_1)\psi_0(\boldsymbol{x}_1, \dots \boldsymbol{x}_N)\rangle] = 0$$

$$\dots (5.9)$$

Where we have used the fact that $\psi_0(H)$ is antisymmetric (symmetric) under interchange of the x_i. In (5.9), E is the total energy. Assuming that the electron is incident with momentum p_0 in the state ϕ_0,

$$E = \frac{p_0^2}{4} + E_0 + \varepsilon_0 \qquad \dots (5.10)$$

Here, we have taken ε_0 to be the average (Hartree-Fock) energy of the state ψ_0, i.e. $\varepsilon_0 = \langle\psi_0|H_A|\psi_0\rangle$. Using equation (5.1) and (5.6), (5.9) becomes

$$(\nabla_{R_0}^2 + p_a^2)G_a(\boldsymbol{R}_0) = 4\sum_{a'} U_{aa'}(\boldsymbol{R}_0)\,G_{a'}(\boldsymbol{R}_0) - 4\sum_{a'} \int L_{aa'}(\boldsymbol{R}_0, \boldsymbol{R}_1)G_{a'}(\boldsymbol{R}_1)\,d\boldsymbol{R}_1$$

$$\dots (5.11)$$

where

$$p_a^2 = p_0^2 + 4(E_0 - E_a) \qquad \dots (5.12)$$

Solving the coupled equations (5.11) subject to the boundary condition

$$G_a(\mathbf{R}_0)_{R_0\to\infty} = e^{ip_0.\mathbf{R}_0}\,\delta_{a0} + g_{0a}(\widehat{\mathbf{R}}_0)\frac{e^{ip_a.R_0}}{R_0} \qquad \text{.... (5.13)}$$

yields the scattering amplitude g_{0a} for the electron transition $\phi_0 \to \phi_a$ and hence the differential cross section

$$\frac{d\sigma_{0a}}{d\Omega} = \frac{p_a}{p_0}|g_{0a}|^2 \qquad \text{.... (5.14)}$$

and total cross section is

$$\sigma_{tot} = \Sigma_a\,\sigma_{0a} \qquad \text{.... (5.15)}$$

5.3 RESULT AND DISCUSSION

We have used equation (5.14) to calculate inelastic differential scattering cross sections (DCS) of Krypton by electron impact at different *viz* energies 20, 15,13.5 and 12 eV. Also to obtain total scattering cross section for 5s state of Krypton we have used equation (5.15).

5.3.1   5s[3/2] EXCITATION

Figure (5.1) represents the present calculation of DCS of Krypton by electron impact by 20 eV electron impact energy. For comparision purpose we have plotted experimental data of Guo *et al* [15] and theoretical result of Khakoo *et al* [16] using unitarized first order many body theory (UFOMBT). The respective results are represented by P, E and U respectively. From figure, we observe that our results are in good agreement with experimental as well as theoretical results. However our results are towards higher side while other theoretical result U is lower side of experimental data E. But all three curves show the same position of dip that is around 90^0 scattering angle.

Figure (5.2) provide the present results as figure (5.1) but at 15 eV electron impact energy. We are surprised that all three curves showed different angular variation of DCS. We are unable to explain this random feature in either experimental data or theoretical result.

Figure (5.3) and (5.4) presents our results along with experimental data at 13.5 eV and 12 eV respectively. In both the figures the trend of present theoretical results and other available theoretical result is same. However the experimental data provide abrupt DCS.

5.3.2   5s[1/2] EXCITATION

Similar to 5s[3/2] excitation we have plotted the DCS of Krypton of 5s[1/2] excitation in figure (5.5) to (5.8). The electron impact energies are taken similar to those in 5s[3/2] excitation. Further same the comparison is made *i.e.* experimental [15] and theoretical [16]. At all these energies the present results are in reasonable agreement with experimental and theoretical calculation except in figure (5.8) in which experimental values are slightly smaller at lower angles. In these figures we have also observed as impact energy decreases the cross section is also decreased.

5.3.3   TOTAL SCATTERING CROSS SECTION

Figure (5.9) shows the plot of total scattering cross sections of Krypton verses incident electron energy. We have compared our results with available theoretical results of Dasgupta *et al* [17] who have used 51 state R-matrix calculations. From this figure we have observed that till 10 eV energy our results provide reasonable agreement, but after 10 eV the present calculation shows a few resonance peaks. This is a good feature for many applications but to be confirmed by other theoretical results.

5.4 CONCLUDING REMARKS

The present work on electron impact excitation of Krypton is motivated by discrepancies found in previous noble gas atoms. However a very little work has been done on Krypton excitation. The theoretical modeling of electron scattering from the rare gases is difficult because of complexity of representing the role of core electrons. The present role shows clearly a good representation of the target wave function which is frozen core type approximation. These results provide a much more complete picture of electron excitation of such higher noble gas atom.

FIGURE CAPTIONS

Figure [5.1] : **DCS of Kr [3/2] by 20 eV electron impact energy**

—————— : Present result

• • • • : Experimental result of Guo *et al* [15]

— · — ·· — · — ·· : Theoretical result of UFOMBT [16]

Figure [5.2] : **DCS of Kr [3/2] by 15 eV electron impact energy**

—————— : Present result

• • • • : Experimental result of Guo *et al* [15]

— · — ·· — · — ·· : Theoretical result of UFOMBT [16]

Figure [5.3] : **DCS of Kr [3/2] by 13.5 eV electron impact energy**

—————— : Present result

• • • • : Experimental result of Guo *et al* [15]

— · — ·· — · — ·· : Theoretical result of UFOMBT [16]

Figure [5.4] : **DCS of Kr [3/2] by 12 eV electron impact energy**

—————— : Present result

• • • • : Experimental result of Guo *et al* [15]

— · — ·· — · — ·· : Theoretical result of UFOMBT [16]

Figure [5.5] : **DCS of Kr [1/2] by 20 eV electron impact energy**

—————— : Present result

• • • • : Experimental result of Guo *et al* [15]

— · — ·· — · — ·· : Theoretical result of UFOMBT [16]

DCS OF KRYPTON 5s (3/2) BY 20 eV ELECTRON IMPACT ENERGY

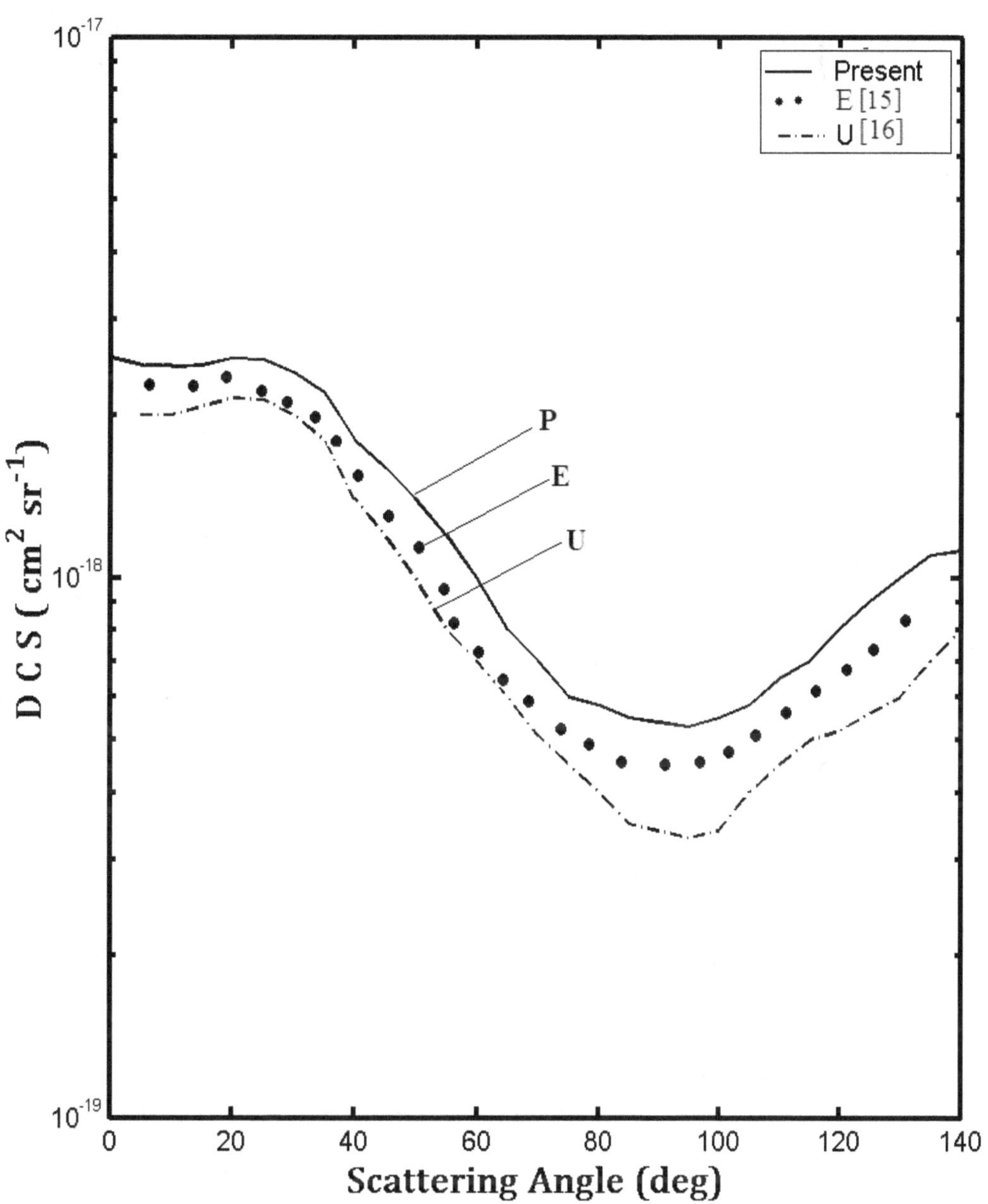

FIGURE [5.1]

DCS OF KRYPTON 5s (3/2) BY 15 eV ELECTRON IMPACT ENERGY

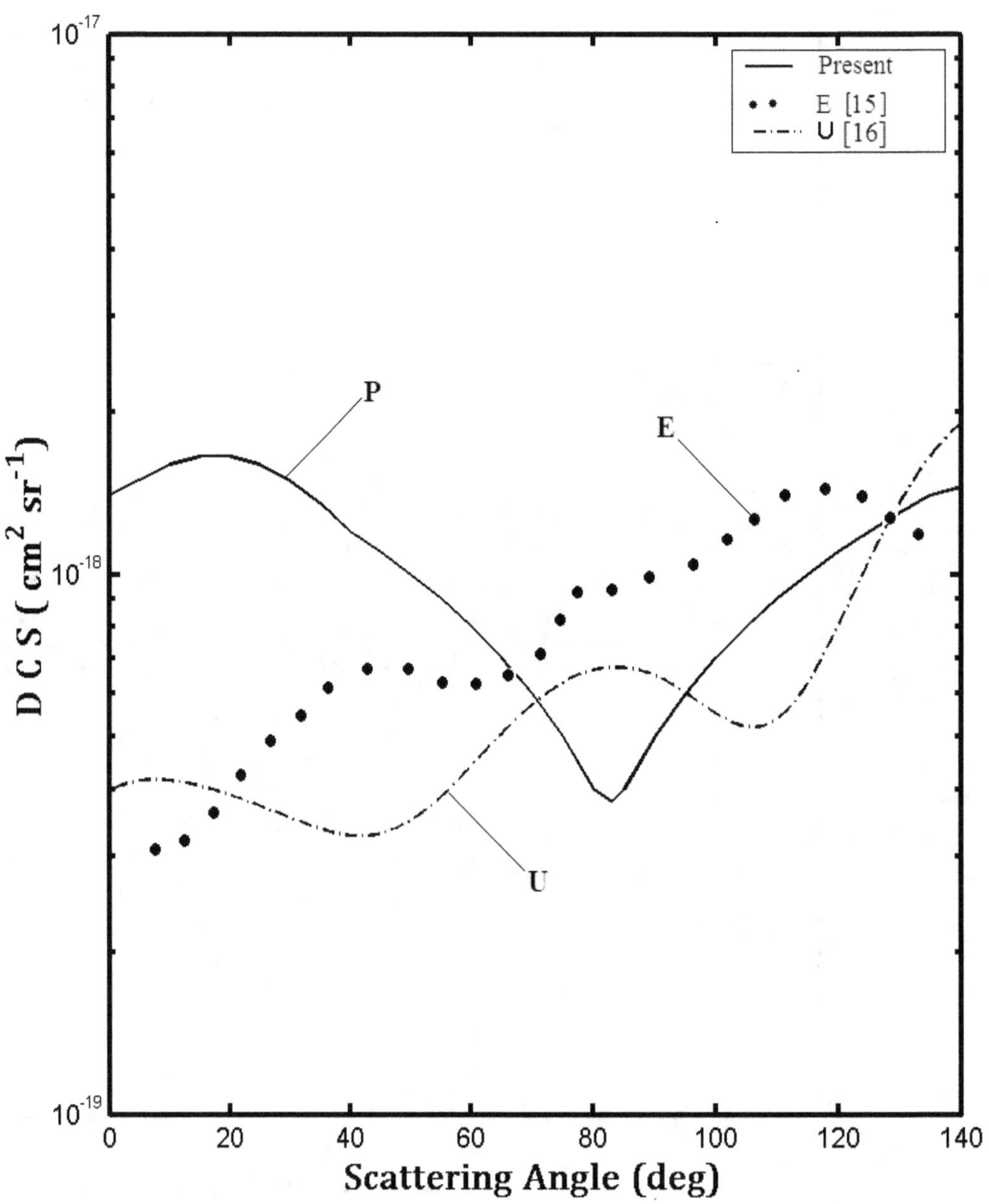

FIGURE [5.2]

Present
E [15]
U [16]
10⁻¹⁷
10⁻¹⁸
10⁻¹⁹
P
E
U
DCS (cm² sr⁻¹)
Scattering Angle (deg)
0
20
40
60
80
100
120
140

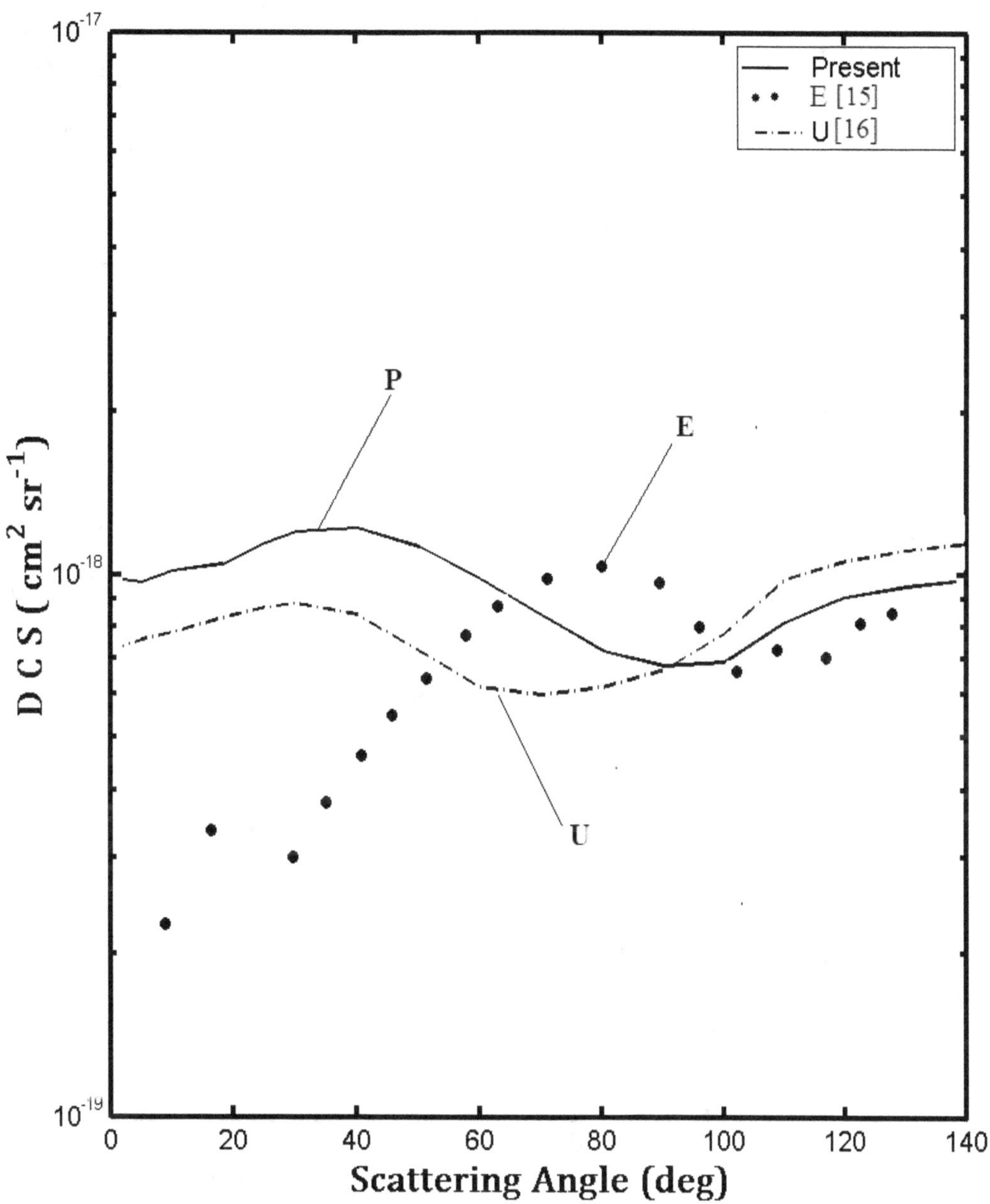

FIGURE [5.3]

DCS OF KRYPTON 5s (3/2) BY 12 eV ELECTRON IMPACT ENERGY

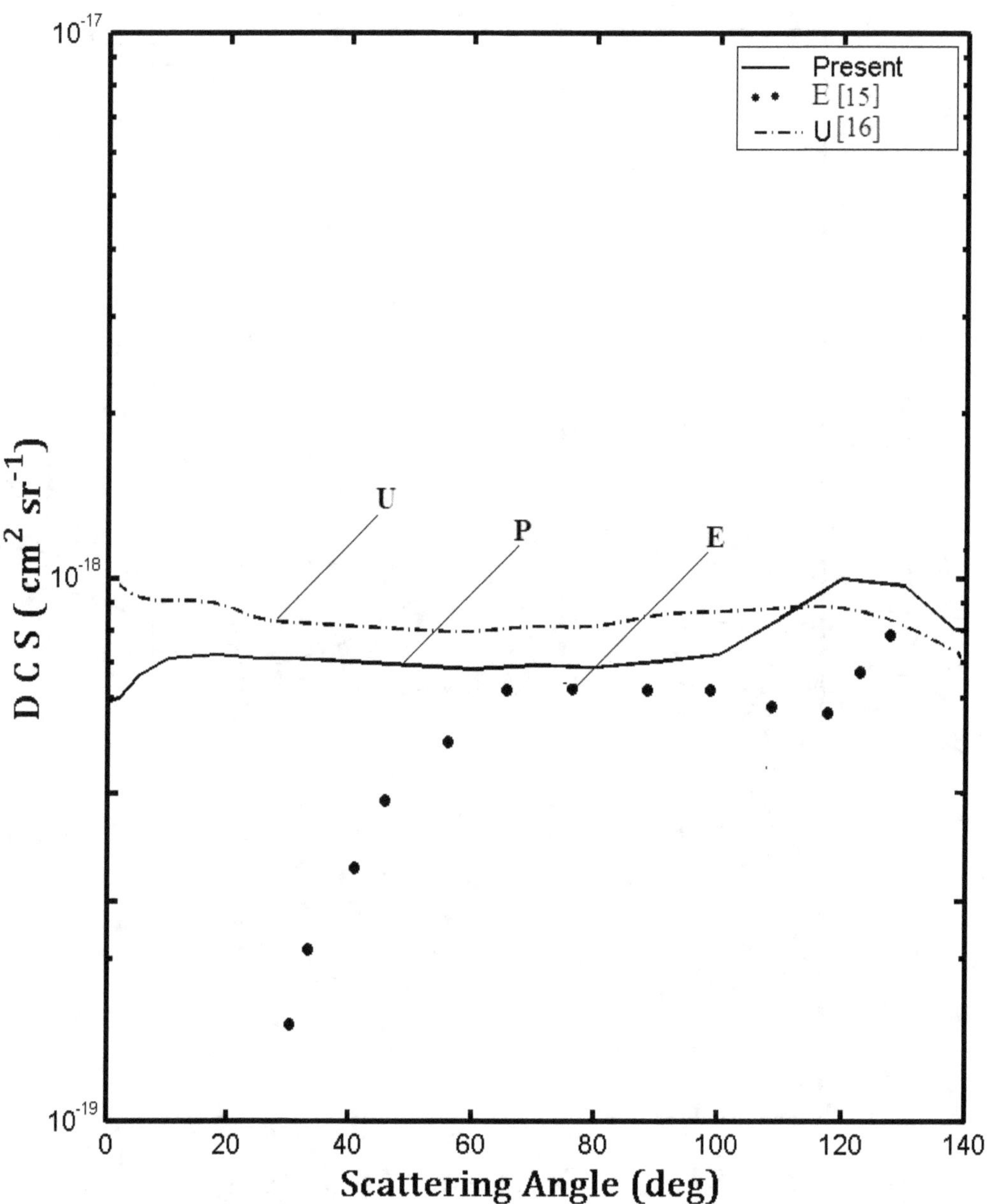

FIGURE [5.4]

DCS OF KRYPTON 5s (1/2) BY 20 eV ELECTRON IMPACT ENERGY

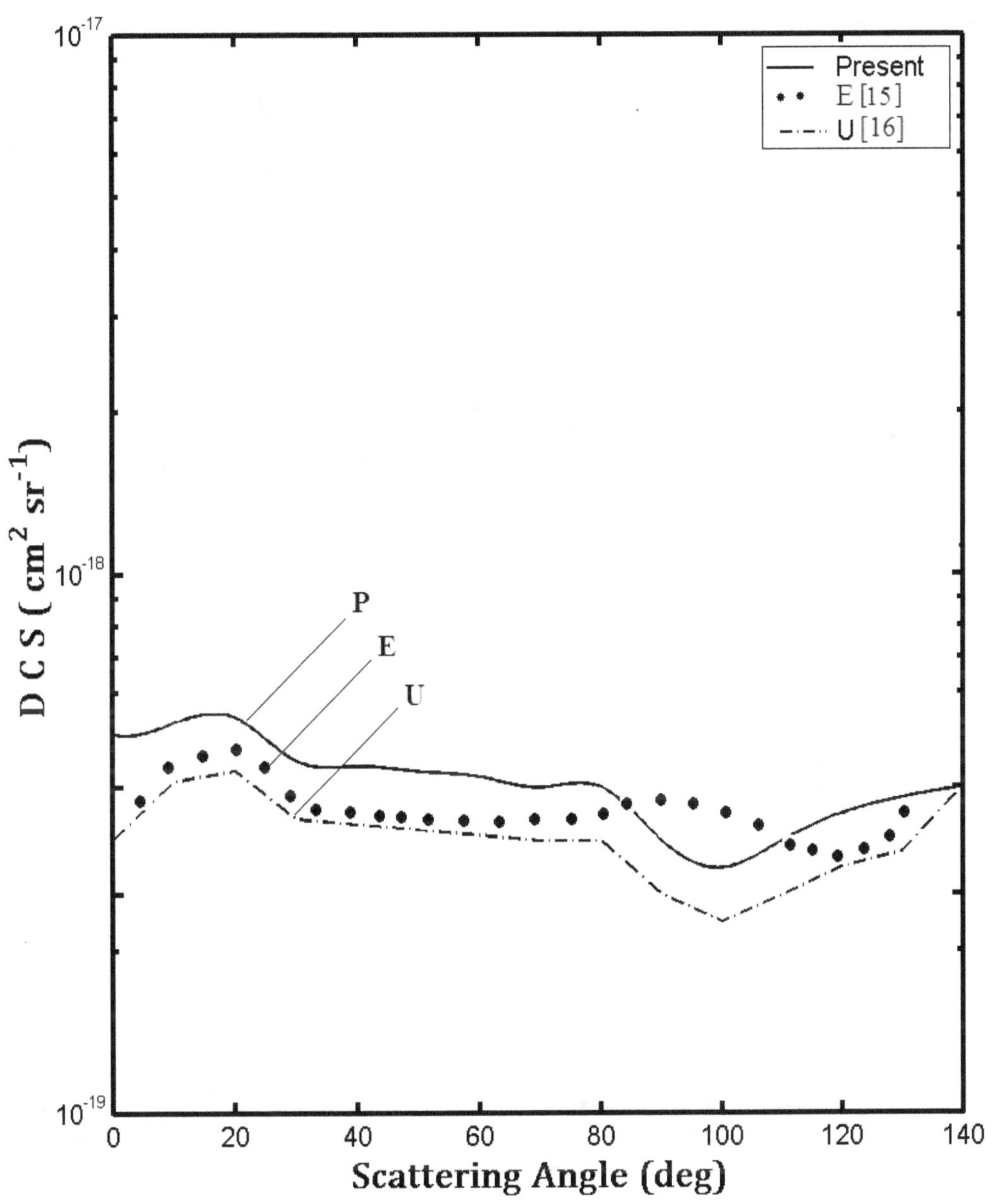

FIGURE [5.5]

DCS OF KRYPTON 5s (1/2) BY 15 eV ELECTRON IMPACT ENERGY

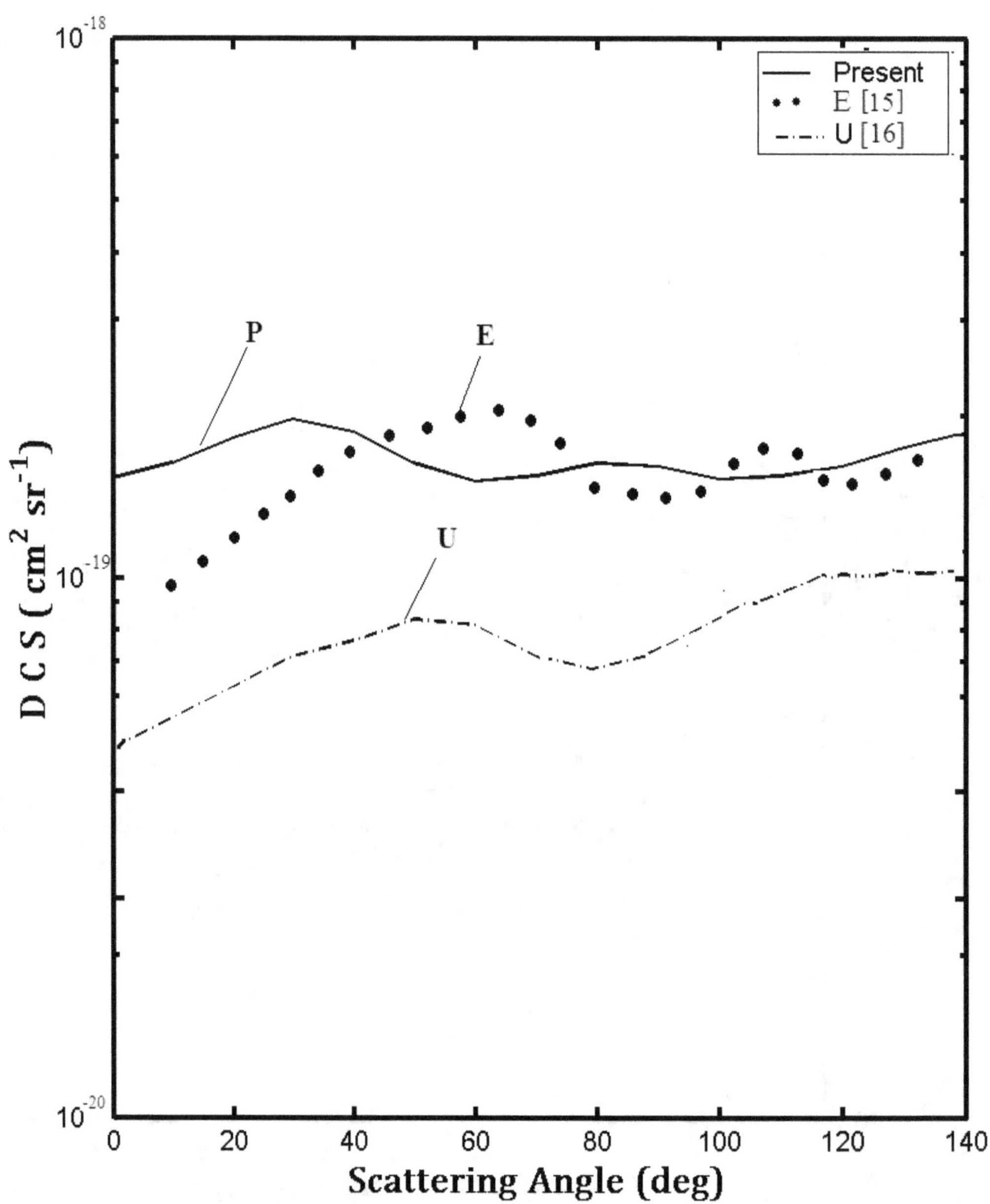

FIGURE [5.6]

DCS OF KRYPTON 5s (1/2) BY 13.5 eV ELECTRON IMPACT ENERGY

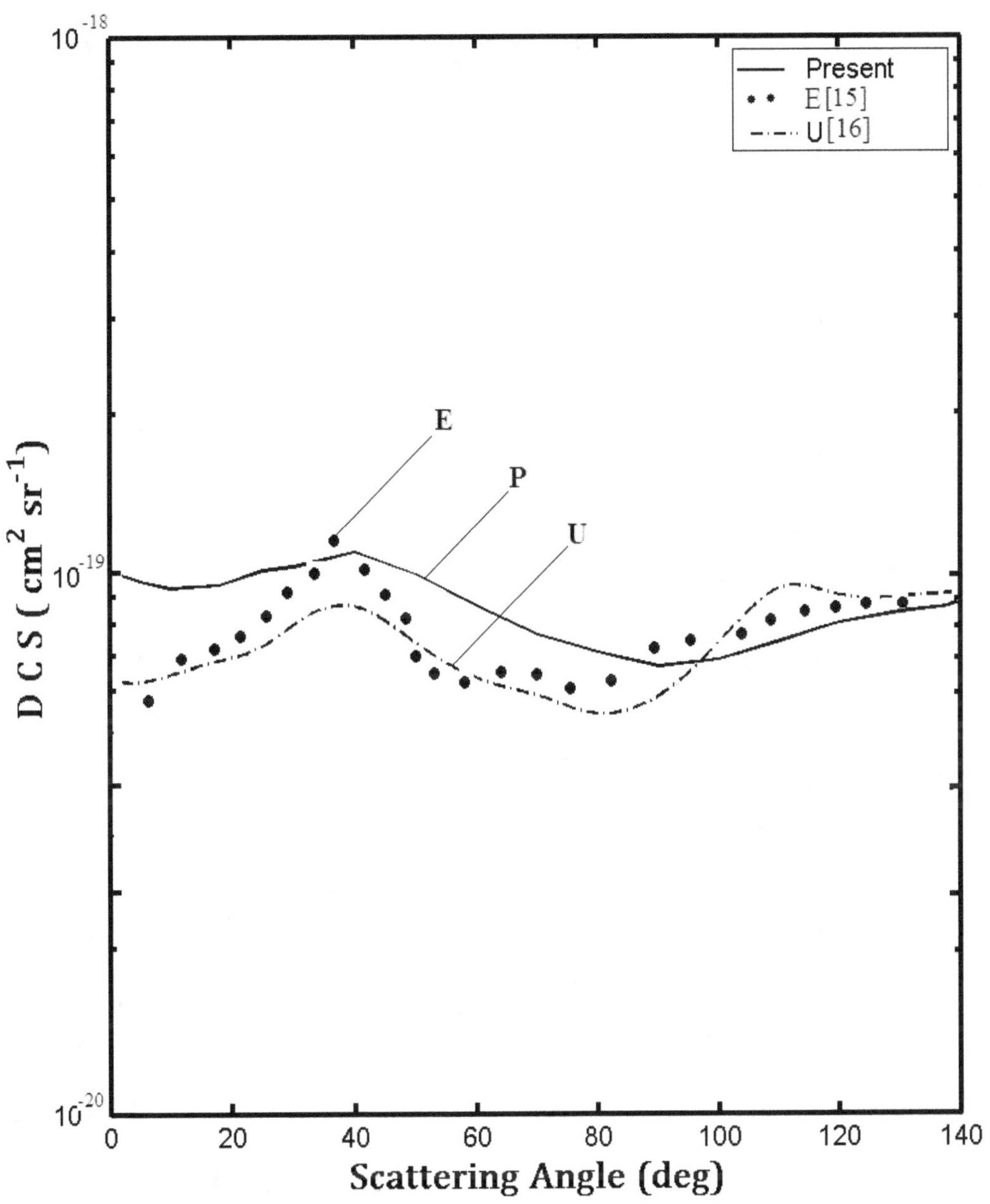

FIGURE [5.7]

DCS OF KRYPTON 5s (1/2) BY 12 eV ELECTRON IMPACT ENERGY

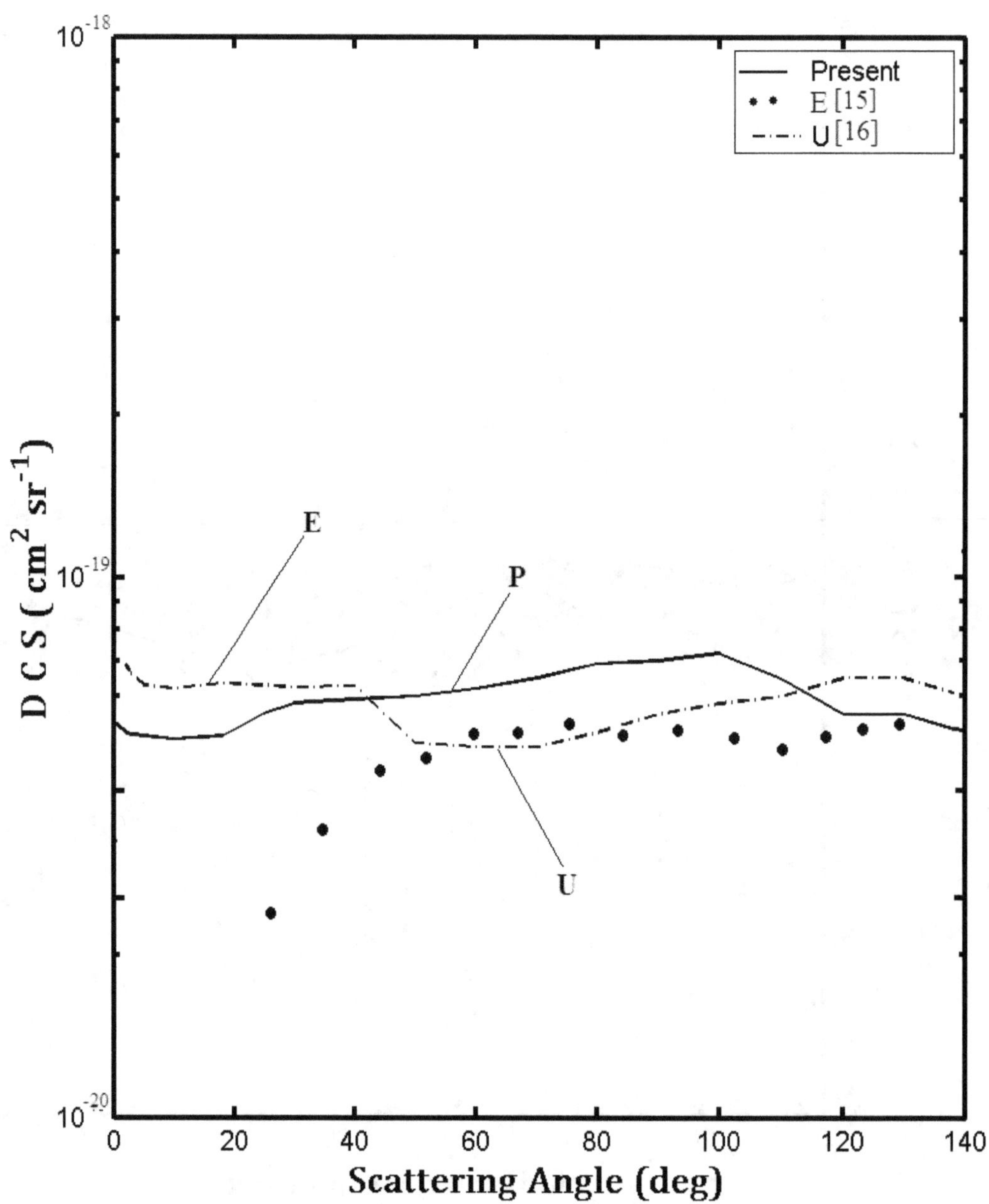

FIGURE [5.8]

TOTAL SCATTERING CROSS SECTION OF KRYPTON

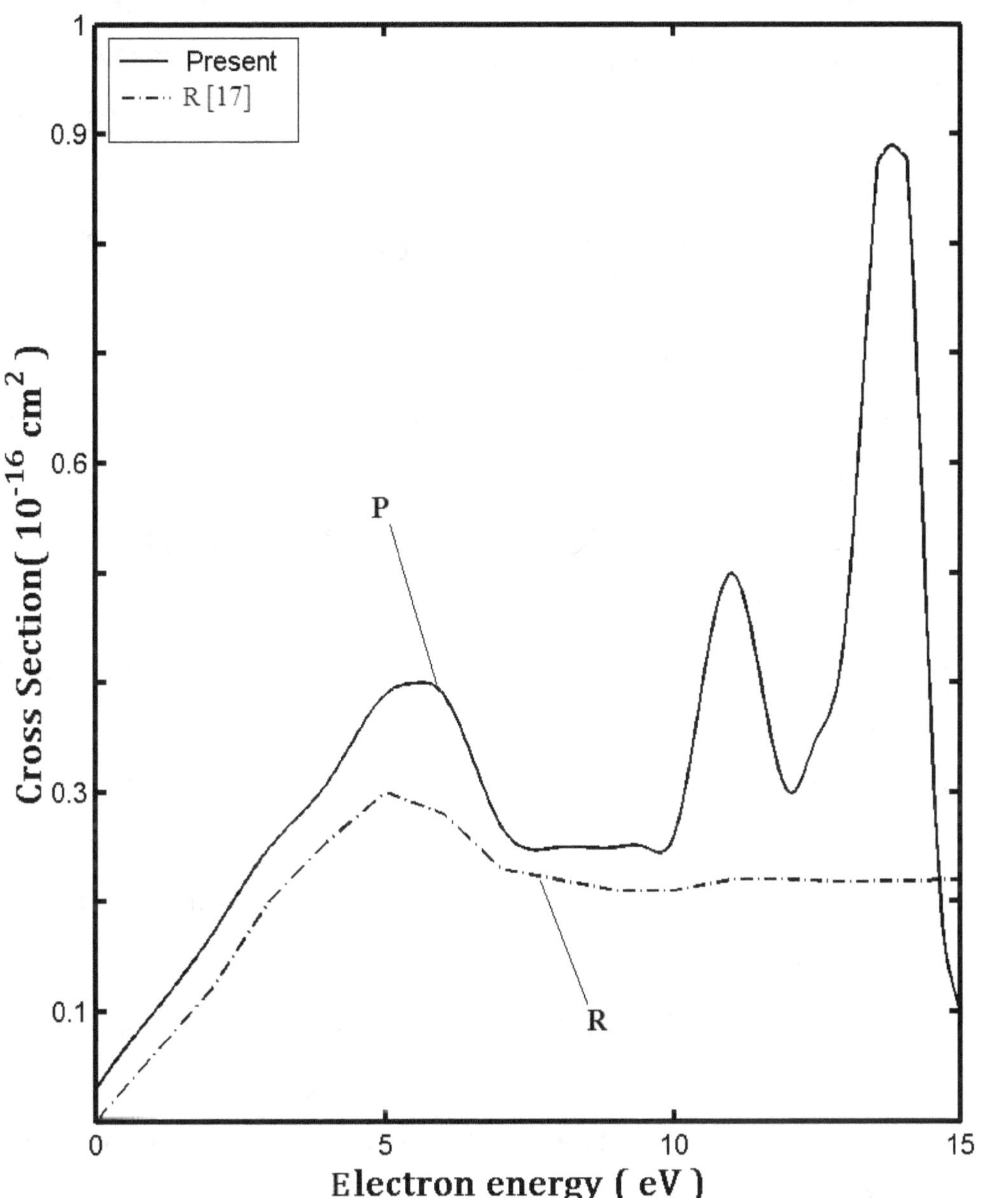

FIGURE [5.9]

REFERENCES

1. R. P. McEachran and A. D. Stauffer, J. Phys. B: At. Mol. Opt. Phys. **36**, 3977 (2003).

2. W. M. Ariyasinghe and C. Goains, Phy. Rev. A **70**, 052709 (2004).

3. J. Zeng, J. Wu, F. Jin, G. Zhao, and J. Yuan, Phy. Rev. A **72**, 042707 (2005).

4. R. O. Jung *et al,* Phys. Rev. Lett. **94**, 163202 (2005).

5. K. Bartschat and O. Zatsarinny, J. Phys. B: At. Mol. Opt. Phys. **40,** F43–F49 (2007).

6. Dummler *et al, J. Phys. B: At. Mol. Opt. Phys.* 28, 2985(1995).

7. S. Chen, R. P. McEachran and A. D. Stauffer, J. Phys. B: At. Mol. Opt. Phys. **41** 025201 (2008).

8. I. Yu Kretinin, A. V. Krisilov and B. A. Zon, J. Phys. B: At. Mol. Opt. Phys. **41** 215206 (2008).

9. D. C. Griffin and C. P. Balance, J. Phys. B: At. Mol. Opt. Phys. **42**, 235201 (2009).

10. O. Zatsarinny and K. Bartschat, J. Phys. B: At. Mol. Opt. Phys. **43**, 074031 (2010).

11. T. H. Hoffmann, M-WRuf, H. Hotop, O. Zatsarinny, K. Bartschat and M. Allan, J. Phys. B: At. Mol. Opt. Phys. **43**, 085206 (2010).

12. I. Linert, B. Mielewska, G. C. King and M. Zubek, Phys. Rev. A **81**, 012706 (2010).

13. M. Allan, O. Zatsarinny and K. Bartschat, J. Phys. B: At. Mol. Opt. Phys. **44**, 065201 (2011).

14. E. Clementi and C. Roetti, At. Data Nucl. Data Tables **14**, 177(1974).

15. Xuezhe Guo *et al*, J. Phys. B: At. Mol. Opt. Phys. **33**,1895(2000).

16. M. A. Khakoo *et al*, J. Phys. B: At. Mol. Opt. Phys.**32**, L155 (1999).

17. A. Dasgupta, K. Bartschat, D. Vaid, A. N. Grum-Grzhimailo, D. H. Madison, M. Blaha, and J. L. Giuliani, Phys. Rev. A **64**,052710 (2001).

CHAPTER - 6

SUMMARY, APPLICATIONS AND FUTURE ASPECTS

6.1 SUMMARY

The theoretical research of electron and positron impact excitation with atoms is entering a new phase in the atomic world. Many of the important atomic excitation functions have been surveyed again and again in semi-relativistic and relativistic quantum mechanical approach. There are so many points to more work of this type especially for inert atoms due to immense use and technology available to support relative outcomes of excitation functions. The complete thesis is an author's attempt to understand and solve the mysteries of the elastic and inelastic scattering of the charged particles with atomic target as inert atoms. In this sequence the work theme of the thesis has been segregated in to six well defined chapters. Knowing the importance of the introduction we have given a proper place to it in the first chapter. After a brief of the preliminary remark about collision physics and put forward the basic idea about the methodology and application of the scattering in the various fields of science and technology , what motivated to study such topic and what is the role of such study in the field of science have been discussed. We have studied various scattering parameters used in the study of atomic collision and approximation methods of scattering parameters. Hopefully, in this thesis we have included the most important collisional parameters like differential scattering cross section (DCS) and total scattering cross section (TCS) for Helium, Neon, Argon and Krypton.

In second chapter we have taken Helium which provides testing ground for theoretical and experimental methods for evaluating the validity of collision theory as a three-electron system. We have calculated differential scattering cross section (DCS) for ground state excitation of atomic Helium at various energies of electron impact using outcome of the Pseudostate Close Coupling method with a non-orthogonal-L^2 basis. Also, we have computed total scattering cross sections (TCS) of Helium using same theory. On comparing our results by other available theoretical and experimental results for electron impact excitation of Helium atom at same impact energies, our results has been found in agreement showing the better inviolability of terms used in the calculations. In third chapter, keeping in mind the immense use of the Neon such as in scintillation counters, neutron fission counters, proportional counters, and ionization chambers for detection of charged particles, gas lasers, antifog devices, electrical current detectors, and lightning arrestors *etc*, we have focused our attention on elastic and inelastic electron impact excitation of Neon. Elastic differential cross section (DCS) has been calculated by the use of radial Dirac equations which includes phase shift. Related phase shift is calculated by Hartree-Fock (DHF) type potential. The related potential is simplified by using Buhring's power series method based on a cubic-spline interpolation of the potential function. For inelastic scattering, we have considered the distorted wave Born approximation (DWBA) theory for electron impact excitation of atoms. In fourth chapter, we have taken Argon which is most ubiquitous noble gas of the earth's atmosphere. Elastic differential scattering cross sections (DCS) have been calculated by the scattering of electrons and positrons from Argon atom and result is described by a potential scattering model containing the static and polarization interactions between the incident particle and the target plus exchange in the case of electrons. For each impact energy the phase shifts of lower partial waves are obtained exactly by numerical integration of radial wave equation. The Born approximation is used to obtain contribution of higher partial waves to the scattering amplitude. Evermore for inelastic scattering we adopt Born-Hartree-Bethe approximation taking the completeness property of atomic wavefunction. Calculation of TICS, under the frame work of first Born approximation involving only ground state wavefunction that requires no adjustment parameter, are also done in this chapter.

The fifth chapter is devoted to study of Krypton in which we have focused our study on calculation of differential and total scattering cross section of 5s [3/2] and 5s[1/2] excitation states of Krypton at low projectile energies of electron using the Hartree-Fock wavefunctions. Then we have compared our calculated results with other theoretical as well as experimental data. Present result finds its legitimacy and somewhere quotes the earlier theories and experiments to be evaluated.

The sixth chapter provides a summarizing role of the whole present work of this thesis. The outcome of this present study takes a specified position in the field of science and modern technology. The gravity of the present work can be analyzed by knowing the great importance of collision physics in the field of medical sciences, astrophysics and plasma physics. This work will help noble society of the scientific world. Besides generating the interest in physics, this present study is expected to make more interaction among the people related with atomic collision physics.

6.2 APPLICATIONS OF REPORTED WORK

In fact, anything without its application becomes idle. This natural law is applicable to present work also. In above scenario collision physics put the foundation stone of development and advent of science and technology. Not only the physical sciences and technology but medical science is also taking the advantage of collision theory. In many branches of physics *viz* in the radiobiology, availability of electron and positron cross sections in low-energy range is a condition for accurate particle transport calculations. In medical physics the studies of the DNA damage due to radionuclides attached to the DNA are underway. These radionuclides emit electrons in electron volt energy range. These electrons have stopping ranges below 20 nm and can therefore directly damage the DNA as well as produce free radicals and then damage the DNA due to a secondary chemical step. Also positron emitters have a low-energy part of their spectra and may cause the same effect if they are attached to DNA. The scattering theory plays a significant role and applied in many advanced area of science and technology as radar, remote sensing, medical ultrasound, semiconductor wafer inspection, polymerization process monitoring, acoustic tiling, free space communication and computer generated imagery *etc.* when we move at the age of air transportation then the process of scattering plays a key role in global positioning system (GPS). The theoretical model that describes the power of a scattered GPS signal as a function of geometrical and environmental parameters has been developed. This model is based on a bistatic radar equation derived using the geometric optics limit of the Kirchoff approximation. A transition to satellite altitude, together with satellite velocities, makes the peak power reduction and the Doppler spreading effect a significant problem for wind retrieval based on delay mapping technique. At the same time, different time delays and different Doppler shifts on the scattered GPs signal could form relatively small spatial cells on sea surface, suggesting mapping of the wave slope probability distribution in synthetic aperture radar (SAR). The science of colours of different events depends on the scattering of the light. As the colour of the sky is blue and also everyone can observed the red colour of sun set or rise. The choice of the signal colour (taken as red of danger signals *etc*) depends on scattering processes. This is because the red colour has a long wavelength and hence scatters least. The blue light is almost scattered from the direct coming to own eye from the sun through the air leaving only the red colour seen. On one side of the investigation is that, how laser light is affected by particles randomly suspended in a medium such as smoke, fog or water to determine the distortion in the images. A slight spectral broadening (few MHz) of the forward scattered light is passed by the smoke or fog particles. After passing the light would be bent from their initial scattering angle and produce distortion. From this distortion, we measure the temporal coherence of the scattered light. But on the other side the small angle approximation (SSA) to the radiative transport equation is widely used in predicting the image quality for remote sensing application. An investigation is undertaken to determine the range of applicability of the SSA. In the first set of experiments, various size of polystyrene spheres suspended in water are used as a scattered medium. Then the volume scattering function (VSF) sometimes called scattering phase function is calculated from the Mie theory and is measured directly. The VSF is then used as input to SSA and the point spread function (PSF) is calculated. On the basis of PSF, we can measure the thickness of the cloud in the sky and weather prediction parameters.

First target used in the present work is Helium. It is unique and special because it plays a vital role in various fields. Helium is lighter than air due to this, airships and balloons are inflected with it for lift. It is used as a protective gas in growing silicon and germanium crystals. Helium is used to cool the superconducting magnets in modern MRI scanners. The use of Helium reduces the distorting effects of temperature variation in the space between lenses in some telescopes. On account of the above use, we can say that Helium is much profitable for human beings. In nuclear physics, Helium ions or alpha particles serve as projectiles in bombarding heavy nuclei to produce energy or to obtain artificial radioisotopes. It is also used for heat transfer and coolant in nuclear reactors. Some other applications of Helium scattering include: detecting leaks in pressure containers and high-vacuum equipment; in lasers; in luminous signs for advertising; to fill space between lenses in optical instruments non-reactively; to provide an inert atmosphere for chemical reactions in the absence of air; to displace fuels and oxidizers from storage tanks in rockets or to introduce fuels into combustion chambers under Helium pressure; as a non-nitrogen diluent for oxygen in SCUBA diving (so divers avoid the bends); and to mix with oxygen for treatment of respiratory diseases. Moreover from research point of view electron collisions with Helium atoms are most important and are the subject of much study. Experimentally, Helium is inert and easy to work with. From a theoretical standpoint, it is the simplest atom for which there are no exact wave functions or atomic potentials. Consequently, this collision system is a testing ground for theoretical and experimental methods before subsequent application to more complex systems.

The second target used in this reported work is Neon. After Hydrogen, Helium, Oxygen and Carbon, Neon gas is the fifth most abundant element in the universe but its presence is rare on Earth. A large amount of Neon is produced during volcanic eruptions. Unlike other inert gases, Neon discharges electricity even at normal current and voltages. Neon gas, filled in a tube, produces a bright orange-red colored light, when electric current is passed through the tube under a low pressure condition. The characteristic discharge property of Neon is used in fluorescent lamps, Neon glow lamps (or simply Neon lamps), and various other lighting systems. Such lamps can be operated even at low voltages. Due to its wide applications in outdoor advertising displays and lamps, Neon is also referred to as fill gas. If mercury is added in trace quantities, the orange-red light turns into a brilliant blue color. By changing the composition of Neon and Mercury, various color shades of light can be created. Such lighting effects are extensively used in the interior designing of house and/or landscaping. One of the major applications of Neon gas is in the advertising signs and/or displays also called Neon signs. Operating at high voltages (2 kilovolts and more), Neon signs were discovered for the first time in early 20th century. Since then, this inert gas has been used in manufacturing advertising signs worldwide. Neon light has the ability to penetrate fog, in which other lights are impossible to detect. Hence it forms a valuable lighting system in the extreme cold climatic regions. This property of Neon light is also applied in airplane or aircraft beacons. Recently it is seen that fluorescence enhancement in an ultraviolet plasma grating is limited by ionization potential of Neon atoms. This limitation by high speed electrons impact by Neon requires much deep demonstration. So it becomes necessary to know role of collision and collisional parameters of Neon by electron impact. A mixing of the buffer gas with relatively low ionization potential increases intensity of fluorescence emission by order of magnitude with respect to that from pure Neon atom. Argon which has relatively low ionization potential than Neon can full fill this requirement of ultraviolet grating spectra. Neon serves as a potential cryogenic refrigerant in the liquid state. According to chemical studies, it is revealed that per unit volume of liquid Neon has 40 times refrigerating capacity than that of liquid Helium and three times than liquid Hydrogen. In simpler terms, the latent heat of vaporization of Neon is three times more than that of hydrogen and 40 times than that of Helium. In combination with Helium gas, Neon is used to make Helium-Neon lasers. While conducting the researches for atomic particles, Neon gas is used in trace amounts for preparing the spark chamber mixtures. Some other Neon uses include lightning arrestors, gaseous conduction lamps, wave meter tubes, television tubes, vacuum tubes, and high-voltage testers. Neon is also used in small plasma displays such as personal digital assistants (PDAs) and cell phones.

Argon is the third target used in present thesis because of its wide applications in metallurgy, cryogenic, electronic, laboratory and as light sources. It is used in low pressure gas discharge tubes as a filler gas, emitting bluish light. It is also mixed with other inert gases in Mercury and Sodium vapor lamps. In metallurgy it is used to shield and protect welding metal arcs; in surface cleaning of metals; as a working fluid in plasma arc devices; as an inert blanket in melting and casting of certain alloys; to atomize molten metals and produce their powder; and in high temperature soldering and refining operations and powder metal sintering. In the laboratory, Argon is used as a carrier gas for gas chromatography; or for metal analysis by furnace atomic absorption or inductively coupled plasma emission spectrophotometry; and as a filler gas (often mixed with other gas) in Geiger–Muller, proportional cosmic ray and scintillation counters. It is also used as inert atmosphere in glove boxes to carry out reactions and handling of air sensitive substances. Argon is used as a low-temperature cryogenic fluid for isothermal baths. It is also used in air sampling by condensing the air in a trap and subsequently analyzing organic pollutants. In electronic industry Argon and

Helium are used as protective atmosphere and heat-transfer medium to grow single crystals of ultrapure semiconductors; and as diluents and carriers of dopant gases such as phosphine or arsine. Argon is also used in multi-species actionometry to study the dissociation fraction of a molecule such as nitrogen by comparing the emission lines from these gases. In case of optical emission spectroscopy of discharge plasma with known concentration of inert gases, Argon can be used to determine the concentration of reactive species such as atomic fluorine. Some of the Argon transitions are in the 395–470 nm range and are useful for optical emission spectroscopy plasma diagnostics. In addition, optical emission spectroscopes of similar transitions have been used to estimate the number densities of argon atoms in the $3p^54s$ metastable and resonance states. More generally, cross sections for these transitions are important in computer models of low temperature plasma conditions where the metastable populations can be large.

Lastly we have considered the Krypton as atomic target in the present work due to its immense use in the field of science and technology. Krypton is used in halogen sealed beam headlights to increase light output by allowing thinner filaments to be used with acceptable useful lifetimes. It is also used in lasers, in particular mixed with fluorine to create an 'excimer' mixture that is a precursor to a molecule which exists in the excited state but not in the ground state. In excimer lasers, the gas mixture is pulsed to form short lived molecules to release the energy by emission of light. Krypton emits a brilliant white light when electrified this is why it is used in photographic flash equipments. Other applications of Krypton are sterilization of fluids and lithographic fabrication of semiconductors. Emission lines arising from transitions in ions of Krypton are increasingly being used for diagnosing tokamak fusion plasmas, as well as being observed in a variety of other high temperature plasmas. Additionally, diagnostic experiments for several Krypton ions are in progress because spectral line intensity ratios, particularly in the XUV region, may be useful in diagnosing alpha particles produced in burning DT plasma.

6.3 FUTURE ASPECTS OF PRESENT WORK

Electron (positron)-atom scattering data are essential in the analysis of important physical phenomena in many scientific and technological areas. These include the development of environmentally safer alternatives to replace mercury vapour lighting, laser-produced plasmas as sources for next-generation nanolithography tools, the understanding of atmospheric processes, diagnosis of impurities in fusion plasmas and the quantitative interpretation of astrophysical data. In addition laser ignited fusion, astrophysics experiments in laboratory, opacity measurements, laser excited hollow atoms and atoms in strong magnetic fields requires detailed calculations of atomic scattering data. Despite the great importance of these applications in the sky of scattering world, a little accurate collisional (theoretical or experimental) data is available for many complex atoms and ions. Particularly this is also the case for electron impact excitation and ionization at intermediate energies near the ionization threshold. So, accurate computation of much of the data required in above mentioned field still presents huge computational challenges, even on the latest generation of high performance computers. Moreover multiple scattering faces reduced cross section considering the other traditions of atoms open the new window for the research work to take this study more refined in the area of nanotechnology. It will not be hyperbole to say that seed of new technology will nurture in the field of present work that is collision physics.